Praise for *Friends with the Scale*

Friends with the Scale may be Linda's best work yet (and that's saying a lot!) The examples and strategies she gives are universal to all dieters, but don't be surprised if you often pause and think "That's totally me" and get the feeling the book was written specifically for you!
Chris Dziewulski, Owner/Operator www.StartYourDiet.com

A must read for every dieter who has ever had a love/hate relationship with the scale. Linda's practical tips make the weight-loss journey easier and more fun. I highly recommend this book to all of our clients!
Lynn S. Allen, Director, Quick Weight Loss Centers of Florida
www.QuickWeightLoss.net

Linda Spangle presents a very practical, realistic way to utilize the scale in reaching weight-management goals. *Friends with the Scale* also provides concrete tools on how to move the scale when your weight loss stagnates.
Sandy Livingston, RD, LD/N www.PalmBeachNutritionist.com

In *Friends with the Scale*, Linda Spangle presents "how to" strategies that will allow us to finally use the innocent bathroom scale as the helpful tool it was intended to be. This book will be required reading for all my clients.
Cookie Rosenblum, MA, Weight-Loss Coach
www.RealWeightLossRealWomen.com

Since 1948, TOPS Clubs has been supporting thousands of members' understanding that they are far more than a number on a scale and that the scale is one of many tools that may be used in the weight-loss journey. We applaud the techniques illustrated in *Friends with the Scale* for maintaining a healthy perspective as we work toward our best health.
Barbara Cady, President of TOPS Clubs, Inc. www.tops.org

Linda Spangle has given us ways to positively use our bathroom scale to navigate the challenges of losing weight. She provides a full arsenal of strategies and tools that are essential to conquer and succeed!
Laura C., Coaching client, Fredericksburg, OH

This book provides unique, essential information to assure success with any weight-loss plan or weight maintenance. I'll be recommending it to my patients as well as using the tools personally.
Dr. Bethany Wallace, Denver, CO

FRIENDS
with the
SCALE

Linda Spangle

ALSO BY LINDA SPANGLE

100 Days of Weight Loss
Life Is Hard, Food Is Easy
Success in a Shaker Jar

A Weight Loss Power Guide

FRIENDS
with the
SCALE

HOW TO TURN YOUR SCALE
INTO A **POWERFUL**
WEIGHT LOSS TOOL

Linda Spangle, RN, MA

SunQuest
Media

Published in Denver, Colorado, by SunQuest Media.

SunQuest Media titles may be purchased in bulk for educational, business or sales promotional use. For information, please email Linda@WeightLossJoy.com or call 1-800-298-3020.

Visit us at www.WeightLossJoy.com

Manufactured in the United States of America

10 9 8 7 6 5 4 3

Publisher's Cataloging-In-Publication Data
(Prepared by The Donohue Group, Inc.)

Spangle, Linda, author.
    Friends with the scale : how to turn your scale into a powerful weight loss tool / Linda Spangle, RN, MA.

        pages ; cm.

    "A weight loss power guide."
    ISBN: 978-0-9767057-1-0
    Issued also as an ebook.

    1. Weight loss--Psychological aspects. 2. Weight loss--Popular works. 3. Scales (Weighing instruments) in weight loss. I. Title.

RM222.2 .S53 2014
613.25

Book design by Deborah Perdue, Illumination Graphics

The following service names mentioned in this book are known to be registered trademarks of their respective companies: Medifast, TOPS, Weight Watchers, Jenny Craig, SlimGenics.

The information contained in this book is not a substitute for medical or psychological counseling and care. All matters pertaining to your physical or mental health should be supervised by a physician or other health-care professional.

❧ CONTENTS ❧

Part Four SCALE BARRIERS

Part Five SCALE FRIENDSHIPS

❦ WELCOME ❧

*I*t's early in the morning, and you've gone to the bathroom and brushed your teeth. Now you step on the scale and smile as you note the number.

Smile? Are you kidding me? If you're like most dieters, that weigh-in is usually an awful moment.

But wouldn't it be great if the scale didn't have any power over your day? What if you felt happy and motivated every morning, regardless of what the scale said? I'd like to help you make that a reality.

By the end of this book, I'm confident you'll have left your scale anger and frustration behind. You'll also have figured out how to view your scale as a friend instead of an enemy. And that subtle change will drastically change your weight-management efforts... forever!

* Confused about whether to keep your scale or get rid of it entirely? Take the scale quiz and permanently settle this question.

* Afraid to step on the scale after holidays or vacations? Use the three-day rule to avoid panicking over a scale reading that's not accurate.

* Avoiding the doctor's office because you'll have to get weighed? Pull out the magic response that allows you to skip getting on the scale almost every time.

It's time to change your negative patterns around the scale. Let this book be your guide to building a friendship that will change your morning weigh-in ritual into one of the most positive moments of your day.

✃ *FREE MATERIALS* ✄

Be sure to download the **free support materials** for this book.

www.FriendsWithTheScale.com

* Tips for how to buy a reliable scale
* Interactive quiz to help you decide whether to keep your scale or toss it
* Interviews with leading experts in the weight-loss field
* Simple spreadsheet that automatically calculates five-day averages
* Guide for developing your lifetime scale plan
* Printable version of *Seven Power Keys for Staying Friends with the Scale*

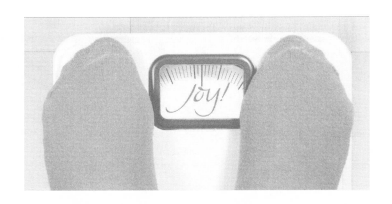

PART ONE

Scale Decisions

CHAPTER 1

What's Wrong with My Scale?

That crazy, stupid piece of metal called a scale! Each morning, you cautiously step on it, hoping for good news. But instead, it tells you that, once again, you have failed.

Your diet didn't work. Your exercise program is useless. And worst of all, you still can't get your dress pants zipped!

In a fit of frustration, you kick the scale as you ask yourself, "What's wrong with it, anyway? Why doesn't the number move? Why can't I ever do anything right?"

But wait! Maybe the scale is saying something entirely different. Perhaps it really wants to tell you about a few things you have no control over.

You got off an airplane last night, which accounts for about three pounds. Did you notice that it's raining today? Try turning your rings, and you'll see the humidity has made your fingers puffy. Go look at the calendar, and you'll suddenly remember what your hormones are doing this week.

Don't give up on your goals because of a number on the scale. Instead, realize that your scale is saying a lot of great things about your weight-loss efforts. You just have to know how to listen.

Turn Your Scale into a Friend

If you're like most dieters, your scale has the ability to change your mood in an instant. In fact, it can even make you feel elated one day and devastated the next.

In an ideal world, your scale would boost your enthusiasm and help you stay on your diet. But it rarely seems to do that. Instead, it routinely destroys your motivation and crushes your self-esteem. Eventually your scale can become your worst enemy, causing you to give up on your weight-loss efforts and head for the refrigerator.

Here's how Susan described her struggle.

Sometimes I'll go a long time without weighing myself. When I finally face reality and get on the scale, I tell myself I'll be fine, no matter what it says. But if my weight is up, I immediately lose my resolve. And as the day goes on, my motivation drops until I start looking for something to eat. Of course, I usually grab stuff that will make me gain even more.

I'm sure you've had similar experiences. When you notice a slight increase in your scale weight, you can't bring yourself to ignore it or let it go. Instead, you immediately turn it into a drama that wrecks your entire day.

Over time, you may have developed a love-hate relationship with your scale. See if any of these phrases sound familiar.

Sometimes getting on my scale...

❖ totally ruins my day.

❖ causes me to go off my diet.

❖ makes me feel anxious and worried.

❖ temporarily destroys my self-esteem.

❖ makes me feel angry or depressed.

Instead of hating your scale with a passion, what if you could figure out how to change your relationship with it? Of course, if you've spent a lot of years feeling sabotaged by your scale, the idea of becoming friends with it may seem impossible. But trust me, it can be done, and it's lot easier than you might think.

The Secret Weapon

When you learn to use it the right way, your scale can show you exactly what you want to see. As a result, it can help you get miraculous results with *any* diet or maintenance plan. But this will happen only if you know what works (and what doesn't) when making the scale a significant part of your total program.

In this book, I'll show you how to ditch your long-term frustration with your scale and turn that little instrument into your best weight-loss tool.

You'll be amazed at how easily your scale shifts its response. Before long, it will give you positive feedback on your efforts, increase your motivation instead of crushing it, and prevent the weigh-in panic that sends you to the refrigerator

Power Keys to Help Build Your Friendship

At the end of selected chapters in this book, you'll find "Power Key" statements. These phrases will remind you of all the ways you are changing your thinking as you build a strong friendship with your scale.

The appendix includes a summary page that lists all seven Power Keys. I encourage you to use these statements as building blocks for a healthy, lifetime scale plan.

Let's get started creating your new BEST FRIEND for life!

CHAPTER 2

The Scale Is My Enemy!

*A*fter years of raising kids and working full-time, Judy was finally going on a vacation. Her husband had made all the arrangements, and they planned to leave in a few days for a trip to Florida.

The best part of this vacation was that all the expenses were being paid by her husband's company. The package included seven glorious days in an oceanfront condo, the use of a convertible sports car and a three-day pass to Disney World.

As she left my office a few days before the trip, Judy said, "I can't wait to leave! This is my dream vacation, and I'm so excited I can hardly stand it!"

When she returned a couple of weeks later, I expected a rave review of her trip. But instead, Judy looked depressed. "What's the matter?" I asked. "Did something go wrong on your vacation?"

She hesitated a minute, then finally confessed. "Actually, I was miserable. Every morning I'd get up and look out at those beautiful surroundings, but then I'd wonder what I weighed. Without my scale, I never knew what kind of day to have!"

The Power of the Scale

Do you ever have days when you wake up feeling cheerful, then weigh yourself and immediately turn into a grouch? Or worse yet, do you give up on your diet program because of the number you saw on your scale?

In the same way it ruined Judy's vacation, your scale can become your worst enemy. In fact, you can get so hooked on it that you can't tell anymore whether it's showing the truth or not. Eventually, this little brat will begin to affect your thoughts as well as your behaviors.

You Are Not Alone!

Sherry had a long-term love-hate relationship with her scale and was often angry with it.

> *Whenever I start a new diet, I feel strong and motivated. This usually lasts for a couple of weeks because, as the scale number goes down, I can see that I'm making progress. But when I don't lose, I get angry and frustrated.*
>
> *Pretty soon, I begin to struggle with every aspect of my program. A few years ago, after a week of overeating, I got so upset that I threw my scale against the bathroom wall. Of course, the scale wasn't even hurt, but I had to repaint the wall.*

In reality, Sherry's anger wasn't at the scale. She was frustrated with the way her own actions were causing the scale number to go up.

During times when you've been slipping up on your diet plan, you've probably had this same response. You're actually angry with *yourself* and the way you've been eating. But since this doesn't feel very good, you choose to be angry at the scale instead.

Peggy had developed the habit of using the scale to confirm her failures. She said, "I recently had a terrible day and totally fell off my diet. I knew I had blown it, and the scale validated this."

How sad! Treating your scale like an authoritarian parent does *not* result in weight-loss success. It only confirms your negative thoughts about yourself.

Break Your Pattern

If you routinely experience anger or discomfort with your scale, it's time to learn how to detach yourself from it and stop letting it ruin your life.

After struggling with her scale for many years, Grace created an unusual way to make this switch.

> *I was never at peace with my scale. Each morning I'd wonder which body part was responsible for that stupid number I saw between my toes. Was it my thick waist? Maybe my heavy thighs?*
>
> *Then I'd engage in negative talk that would last all day (and night) until my next weigh-in. The following morning,*

the story would repeat itself. Finally I decided to change what I said to myself each time I got on the scale.

I made a list of positive words that included beautiful, hot, lovely, sexy, perfect, attractive, fine, and adorable. Then I made small cards and printed a positive word on each one.

Every day when I got on the scale, I pulled a card off the stack and read it aloud. It became my mantra for that day. This simple solution has completely changed my relationship with the scale. Even though some of the words feel a little silly, they help set me up for a day that is positive, strong, and self-affirming instead of negative and powerless.

Instead of having your scale be an aggravating, frustrating enemy, let's flip your relationship with it around! With a few simple changes in your thinking, you can turn your scale into a powerful ally in your weight-loss efforts.

Remember, when you let it ruin your day or cause you to eat, the scale wins. To overcome this, focus on self-care and staying on track, regardless of what the scale says.

As I mentioned before, throughout this book, you'll find a number of Power Keys that will help you maintain a friendship with your scale. I encourage you to make these part of your ongoing self-talk around the scale. Here is the first one.

Power Key 1: Never let my scale win!

CHAPTER 3

No More Drama

Suppose you pick up a new diet book that includes a week's worth of menus. As you plan a grocery list for your program, you are horrified to see that Monday's menu contains spinach, which you hate.

Would you throw the book across the room or yell about the stupid meal plan that contained spinach? Of course not. When Monday came, you would substitute a different vegetable and continue to follow the plan.

Discovering you don't like something on your meal plan probably doesn't stress you very much. So why would you throw your scale across the room because you don't like today's number? What if you could just substitute a different response and go on with your day?

Joyce never got very far with her weight-loss efforts. Whenever her scale number went up instead of down, she felt devastated. Her conclusion each time was, "Why bother?" And instead of looking at her recent actions or patterns, she let the scale decide it was time to quit her program.

Your scale is not your enemy! Instead, it's only one of the many tools in your weight-management program. Just like adjusting to a new diet menu, you don't need to let the scale determine whether or not you lose weight. But sometimes, years of habits can get in the way.

Jackie knew she was a slave to her scale. Here's how she described it.

When I was losing weight a few years ago, my husband thought I was becoming obsessed with the scale, so he put it in the trunk of our car. There were many times when I sneaked into the garage on a cold morning, barefooted and wearing only my bathrobe, so I could weigh myself naked. Not my finest moment!

Here's an interesting thought. What if changing your relationship with the scale actually worked? How would it feel to be comfortable and peaceful about your scale reading instead of distraught by it?

Starting today, I want you to eliminate the drama around your scale. Instead, I want you to lay out a scale management program and figure out how to approach this diet tool in a positive light.

Your Personal Scale Plan

As you go through this book, I'll help you rethink every aspect of how you view your scale. One of the first questions we'll look at is whether you should actually use your scale or whether you should throw it away. You'll quickly learn the answer is not the same for everyone.

If you conclude you want to keep your scale, I'll help you decide how often you should get on it. We'll evaluate whether your best approach is to weigh yourself daily or only at intervals. I'll also help you figure out what the scale reading actually means. (It's not always what you think.)

The Scale Trap

If you're like a lot of dieters, your problem with the scale started many years ago. Think back to your first attempt at losing weight. You ate everything on your food list, did lots of exercise, and then ran to the scale to see if your efforts had worked.

In the beginning, your scale appeared to be providing great feedback. Most of the time, the numbers seemed to match your actions, and you felt encouraged to stick with your efforts. In fact, when the scale numbers went down, you celebrated because this proved you were on the right diet plan.

But on days when the number didn't move, or worse yet, it went up, your self-esteem took a beating. At some point, you concluded either something was wrong with *you* or that your diet program had stopped working.

When Carol called me, she sounded extremely upset. "The scale just won't move!" she cried. "How can I be doing everything perfectly and still not be losing weight? What's wrong with me? Why can't I do this right?"

At this point, Carol had lost her ability to be logical around her scale. Instead, she assumed she had a personality defect that was causing her weight to be stuck day after day. She even wondered what she had done to make her scale hate her so much.

Trust me! Your scale doesn't care about your weight-loss efforts. It knows you will hesitantly step on it each morning, then let the numbers determine many aspects of your day, including your confidence level about life. And sometimes, it will cause you to walk away from a really good diet or exercise plan.

Don't get caught up in crazy drama around your scale. Instead, focus on learning how to view your scale as a powerful *tool* that will help you reach and maintain a healthy weight forever.

CHAPTER 4

To Weigh or Not to Weigh?

*O*ver the past years, you've probably heard lots of conflicting advice. Throw the scale away. No, wait! Weigh yourself every day. No, that's not right either. Never weigh yourself at all.

In the field of weight loss, you'll find plenty of controversy about using the scale. Lots of books and program leaders take an extreme approach and say, "Throw it away! Never weigh yourself again." Sometimes, you're told, "The scale is evil, and it will ruin your weight-loss efforts."

Other sources take the opposite view, suggesting you should weigh yourself regularly, perhaps daily. Many researchers encourage dieters to use the scale as a critical part of any weight-loss program as well as during maintenance. In fact, a number of studies have shown that daily weigh-ins, along with a consistent support system, result in the best long-term outcomes.

So which one is correct? Throw the scale away or step on it every day? Actually, this question doesn't have a right or wrong answer, and either of these choices can bring success. It comes down to learning which approach is right for *you* as well as recognizing the behaviors that get you into trouble.

The Scale Quiz

Here is a simple quiz that will help you identify which scale category fits you best. It will also give you a future roadmap for healthy ways to manage your scale.

Based on what you think or do most of the time, respond to each statement with one of the following:

1=Yes   2=No   3=Sometimes

___ The scale determines my mood for the day.

___ My self-esteem is often connected to what the scale says.

___ I take the scale along when I travel.

___ Thoughts about my weight dominate my day.

___ I frequently talk about my weight or my diet plan.

___ I have a history of anorexia or self-starving.

___ I have a history of bulimia, or binge eating, then purging the food.

___ If my weight is up, I exercise a lot more to make it go back down.

___ When my weight goes up, I punish myself with hard-core exercise or an eating binge.

___ I weigh myself multiple times a day.

___ I can't resist stepping on the scale at the gym or in a friend's bathroom.

___ If I see a scale, I feel compelled to get on it.

___ I punish myself verbally or mentally when the scale goes up.

___ I blame the scale for my weight-loss failure or my regaining weight.

___ Frequently the scale reading makes me want to eat more, not less.

Once you complete the quiz, count the number of responses you have in each category. Here's how to interpret your score.

1 = If you have mostly "yes" answers, you may need to throw your scale away.

2 = If you have mostly "no" answers, you can safely keep your scale.

3 = If you have lots of "sometimes" answers, keep your scale and work on changing your approach to it.

Unless you clearly fit into the toss-your-scale category, you can probably retrain yourself around using it. By working on your thoughts and behavior patterns, you can change your response to the scale and learn to manage it in healthier ways.

Changing Your Thoughts

After years of struggling, Cindy was ready to let go of her obsession with her scale and her weight numbers. We worked on a plan for how often she would weigh herself as well as ways to manage her thoughts and fears around the scale.

After she'd been using her new approach for a few months, Cindy called to tell me how it was going.

A few days ago, I got on the scale and saw the number was up a couple of pounds. In the past, I would have panicked and immediately looked for ways to cut more calories out of my day. But fortunately I heard your voice reminding me that it's just a number.

That helped me respond calmly and keep trusting myself and my new approach. Now I know that regardless of what the scale says, I will continue to follow my healthy eating and exercise plan and stay focused on my program.

Your scale's readout doesn't predict your weight-loss success. It's just a *number* that most likely will be different tomorrow. It says nothing about your future or your ability to reach and maintain a healthy weight in the years ahead.

CHAPTER 5

Go Ahead and Toss the Scale

*O*ver time, some people become so enmeshed with the scale that they can't separate themselves from it. Because it dominates their thoughts and beliefs, they completely lose sight of how to use their scale in healthy ways.

If you've tried everything to manage your response to the scale but continue to struggle with it, you may want to consider getting rid of it. In many cases, tossing your scale will solve the angst you experience each time you weigh yourself.

The Scale Runs Your Life

Is your scale the first thing you think about every morning? If so, take a careful look at what happens after you step on it for your morning weigh-in.

Many dieters instantly move from being cheerful and positive to feeling grouchy and upset when they get on the scale. And when they see a disappointing scale reading, it affects their behaviors for the rest of the day.

If you fit in this category, you may also realize that many days, the scale dominates your thinking and ultimately your actions. It also holds the power to ruin your day. Amanda described how she started having struggles with the scale as a teenager:

During my high school years, I weighed myself obsessively, usually getting on the scale several times a day. Of course, the scale always showed that I weighed more than I thought I did, and I usually felt upset about that for the rest of the day.

Even though it made me feel anxious and depressed, I kept up this pattern for many years. Then in my mid-30s, I decided that weighing myself was simply too upsetting, so I stopped entirely. To make sure I didn't go back to my old habits, I donated my scale to a thrift shop and told the owner I didn't want to ever see it again.

The following morning, I got out of bed, and instead of my usual dread of going into the bathroom where the scale had been, I instantly felt a great sense of relief. I was completely comfortable with not knowing my scale weight, and I realized that I had been yearning to feel this way for a very long time.

It's been twenty years since that day, and I haven't weighed myself since then. I think it's like problem drinkers who decide to never allow booze in their homes. Instead of starting each day feeling paranoid, I found that getting rid of my scale helped me feel healthy and confident.

Obsessed with Your Weight

If your weight enters the room before you do, you're probably hung up on the scale. With this level of struggle, you never get away from your thoughts and feelings about your weight. Over time, concerns about what you weigh constantly trickle into your head and dominate many aspects of your day.

Weight-obsessed dieters usually follow a lot of rituals, such as getting on the scale many times a day and even weighing themselves a couple of times at the gym or at other people's homes.

Unfortunately, scale obsession takes a huge toll. Because your friends and family can't get away from hearing about your weight struggle, it begins to harm your relationships and frustrate those in your life. Eventually, friends may avoid you because conversations always seem to circle back to your weight, your diet, and your angst.

Eating Disorders

People who struggle with eating disorders also tend to be overly concerned about what the scale reading says. For example, anorexics spend hours contemplating how to avoid eating. For some of them, the scale becomes a "god" that provides the ultimate reward for their behaviors.

On the other hand, bulimics use the scale to determine if their actions are being effective. They say things such as, "What do I weigh now? Oh my! That's terrible. OK, what do I weigh now after I've thrown up?"

For these people, the scale alternately provides a sense of exhilaration or a feeling of despair. Then depending on what it says, the scale also tells them whether or not their crazy actions are working.

Weighing Multiple Times a Day

When you hop on the scale many times during the day, you aren't using it the way it was intended. First of all, weighing yourself multiple times a day gives you meaningless information. You might think you know how much your bowel movement weighed or how much you gained from eating lunch. But these are only part of the ever-shifting landscape within your body, and they don't accurately reflect your true weight.

Your body is very complex, and it's constantly changing in response to daily functions. There is no measurement tool that tells you exactly what altered in the last hour. And the scale is probably the most inaccurate guide of all.

What the Scale Knows

Brenda struggled a lot with her self-esteem, and getting on the scale usually made it plummet. She said, "My self-worth is always based on what I weigh. And because I never weigh what I want, I don't ever feel like I'm worthy or valuable!"

For many people, it seems the scale doles out judgment about personality defects or moral character. But evaluating your life based on the number on your scale usually backfires. Instead of challenging you to work on your personal growth, it drives you further into dysfunctional thinking.

Overcoming shaming messages from the scale takes a bit of work. If this is a major issue for you, it's probably best to avoid the scale entirely. That way, you eliminate one of the areas where you tear yourself down and reinforce negative beliefs about yourself.

Here's how Theresa worked through her problem with the scale.

> I had been working pretty hard to lose weight and finally thought I'd jump on the scale. When I got out of bed that morning, I was feeling fabulous. For the past several weeks, I'd been working out and eating really well. I was sure I'd lost weight. But NO! The number was up instead of down. How could that be? So I got bummed out. And I ate.
>
> It suddenly dawned on me that I was eating because of the bad mood that stupid number put me in. Right then I decided I was done with the scale. My new goal is to wear clothes that I haven't fit into for a while. When

*my pants fit better, I'm happy because
I know I'm making progress. I love the
fact that I no longer live and die by the
number on the scale.*

The Three-Day Test

Are you still unsure about whether you need to throw away your scale? Here's a simple test that might help you decide. Follow these guidelines for three days in a row:

* Weigh yourself every morning, but only once each day.

* Tell yourself, "It's just a number, and I am NOT my weight."

* Avoid discussing the scale, your weight, or your diet plans.

If you can do this successfully for three days in a row, you can consider keeping your scale. But look carefully at what you did over those days. Did you sneak into the bathroom to weigh again at some point in the day? Was it uncomfortable avoiding discussions about the scale or your diet? Were you able to do the three steps easily, or did you find yourself complaining about the rules?

You don't have to get rid of your scale forever. But if you realize you can't break your negative scale rituals, I suggest you take it out of your life, at least for a while. At some time in the future, you can always re-evaluate the question and consider getting a scale again. On the other hand, if getting rid of your scale made you feel a lot healthier and less obsessed with your weight, assume that you are better off without it.

CHAPTER 6

Keep Your Scale — It's OK

I've always enjoyed driving a bit fast. But some years ago, I got several speeding tickets within a few months. It wasn't my fault! I just know those police officers were hiding and they were out to get me! But when I reached the point when my speeding tickets were putting me at risk of losing my driver's license, I knew I had to change my behavior.

After getting one of the tickets, I decided to go to court and attempt to negotiate the fee and the number of points on my record. Somehow, I was feeling very emotional that day, and when I had a chance to present my case to the district attorney, I fell apart sobbing in his office. After handing me a few tissues, this kind man gave me some wonderful advice.

> *Every day when you get into your car,*
> *pause for a few seconds. As you put on*
> *your seat belt, say to yourself, "I am now*
> *in the car. I am now driving. And I'm*
> *going to stay alert and aware as I drive."*

> *Then regardless of which street or road*
> *you are driving on, notice every one of*
> *the speed zone signs, and make sure you*
> *are staying close to the posted limits.*

This sage advice helped me change my driving patterns overnight. Since then, I've gone years without getting another speeding ticket. But to this day, anytime I'm driving, my speedometer remains one of my most important tools for staying within the speed zones.

If you've had a similar problem with getting too many speeding tickets, I doubt you would hate your speedometer or rip it out of your car. Instead, you would probably keep a close eye on it whenever you are driving.

Think of your scale in the same way. Don't view it as a police officer who gives you a ticket after you've had a bad day. Instead, practice seeing it as a speedometer for tracking what your weight is doing. Use your scale to help you stay on the road and prevent you from racing toward trouble.

A Healthy Relationship

If you've chosen to keep your scale, you simply need to learn how to use it in healthy ways. Here are a few guidelines for building a great friendship with your scale.

❖ **Step on, step off, leave.**
You don't brush your teeth in the morning, then obsess all day wondering if you should brush

them again. With your scale, build a similar routine. At your chosen time of day, get on the scale, note what it says, write it down if you like, then leave the room.

* **Look, record, move on.**
  Suppose you decided to balance your checkbook. Once you had finished, you'd go about your day, hardly remembering the numbers you saw online or in your checkbook register.

  In the same way, treat your scale reading as a number, nothing else. If you are tracking your weight, record it in your journal, calendar, or online program.

  Then go eat a healthy breakfast, take a walk at lunch, and stay away from the TV much of the evening. Eventually, these actions will bring a much better reward than obsessing about the scale's numbers.

* **Note how you're trending.**
  News websites often show a list of the people or topics that are "trending." These links reflect popular online searches and show the latest stories about those people or events.

  Consider viewing your scale weight in the same way. How is it trending lately? As you monitor it over time, your biggest concern is not the daily number but whether it's trending in the right direction.

It's Only Data

You can also think about your scale reading as being like the stock market. Sometimes the price of a stock will go up or down for no apparent reason. If you're monitoring your portfolio, you know that on any given day, or even during a particular week, these changes mean nothing. But over time, they reflect the truth about your finances.

In the same way, the daily number on your scale does not give complete information. The readings only count if they're still the same after a long time. So whenever you get on the scale, remind yourself, "It's only data." Then go about your day, focusing on healthy actions instead of panic.

Also, don't let your scale label you as a "failure" when it comes to losing weight. Remember, your scale is handing out information, not punishment. It provides numbers, but that's all they are—only data, not a reflection of your life. And these numbers are unrelated to personal characteristics such as love, determination, and commitment.

Healthy Scale Thinking

Once you've decided to keep your scale, you'll want to build healthier patterns around it. Here are a few ideas that will protect you from upsets with your scale.

❖ **Don't assume you've gained weight.**
   A jump in the scale number may have nothing to do with your weight. In reality, your body takes a long time to translate food intake into actual fat stores.

So please let go of your guilty thoughts about whether last night's brownie caused you to gain two pounds.

If you know you've eaten an extra-large meal or food that's high in salt, consider skipping your weigh-in for a day or two. This will allow your body to return to a closer-to-normal balance. Either way, remind yourself that one bad evening doesn't translate into a higher weight.

❖ **Detach from the numbers.**

If you get a poor grade on a school mid-term exam, it doesn't mean you've flunked the class. Instead, it provides information about what you need to do before the end of the term.

Treat the scale with the same level of detached interest. Stop mentally chastising yourself on days when your scale's reading doesn't change or the number goes up. Simply notice what it says, monitor or record it, then get back to work on your healthy living plan.

Sometimes it helps to have a standard phrase that you recite to yourself on days when the scale number has bounced around. Consider saying, "That's interesting" or "OK, that's just today's information."

❖ **Stick with your plan.**

One of the quickest ways to let your weight get out of hand is to stop weighing yourself altogether.

Maybe you convince yourself that if you don't look at the numbers, you aren't gaining weight.

Don't ignore your scale because you don't want to see what it says. If you have a history of weight struggles, you need to *stay aware* of your current situation. It's fine to skip weighing yourself for a few days or even a couple of weeks. But at some point, move past your fear, get back on the scale, and update your data.

CHAPTER 7

The Games We Play

*W*hen the scale doesn't give you the results you'd hoped for, do you attempt to make it say what you want? Maybe you jump off quickly and pretend you didn't see the number. Perhaps you get on and off a bunch of times, hoping the readout will change. Or you start playing around with the scale to see if you can trick it into showing a number you want to see.

Dee's Weigh-in Rituals

Dee belonged to a diet program that had weekly check-ins. At noon every Wednesday, she faithfully went to her group meeting and stepped on the scale. Because she was always determined to see the lowest weight number possible, she told me she had developed a list of rituals for her weigh-in day. They included:

❖ No eating or drinking before weigh-in, no matter what time my meeting was.

❖ Wear lightweight summer clothes year-round. (No heavy outfits!)

- ❖ Make sure to put on my lightest underwear.

- ❖ Leave off extra jewelry, such as my watch.

- ❖ Wear thin socks or none at all.

- ❖ Eat very light meals and maybe even no dinner the day before.

- ❖ Leave my pedometer in my purse. (Who knows how heavy those are!)

- ❖ That morning, pee and pee (and hope to go No. 2) prior to my weigh-in.

Over time, Dee's rituals only made her more obsessive about her scale numbers. And she never wanted to admit she was seeking an extreme, unrealistic readout. Even worse, because of the way she ate on all the other days of the week, Dee's weight rarely changed.

Common Scale Games

Dieters are notorious for inventing secret games around the scale, hoping they can trick it into giving them the results they want. I've had clients who were so hooked into scale games that they flossed their teeth or waited to put in their contacts, hoping for a lower reading.

How many of these scale games have you tried? Put a check mark beside any that you've done at some point.

- ❖ Move the scale to different areas on the floor.

- ❖ Weigh yourself several times a day.

- ❖ Hold your breath while on the scale.

❖ Make sure your hair is dry.

❖ Take out your earrings, remove all jewelry.

❖ Go to the bathroom a few times.

❖ Get on and off the scale many times.

If you recognize your own scale games, look at the reality of what they accomplish. Have they brought you a lot more progress with losing weight? Or have you found that, in spite of these crazy efforts to get a different number on the scale, your pants still don't fit? Deep inside, you know these tricks won't ever improve your weight.

When the Scale Gets Mean

Sometimes, instead of providing information, your scale becomes a scolding, punishing parent. On days when there's an upswing in the number, your scale mocks you by creating nasty messages in your head.

❖ It's all your fault. You ate those chips, cookies, etc.

❖ You can't stay on a diet, no matter what.

❖ Why are you so ... weak, stupid, or lazy?

The worst game of all is when you decide to get even with your scale. In fact, some dieters actually punish themselves by doing an eating binge on days when the scale goes up.

Robert frequently used his scale as an excuse for overeating. When the numbers didn't change for a few days, he would say to himself, "Obviously, my diet isn't working, so screw it. I'll show that stupid scale it can't do that to me. I'm just going to have fun and eat whatever I feel like."

How destructive! Beating yourself up because of a simple math number is completely illogical. It's like saying, "It's raining today, so it must be my fault. I'll show the stupid rain! I'll skip my exercise and overeat."

Regardless of what you do, your scale will give you a number. Some days it's not a "warm fuzzy" number, but it's still just a number. You can't magically shift to a different weight by playing games with the scale.

Starting now, let go of any of the games you play with your scale. Remind yourself that the readout is only a number, and you can't trick it into being something else.

Power Key 2: Remember that I can't trick the scale.

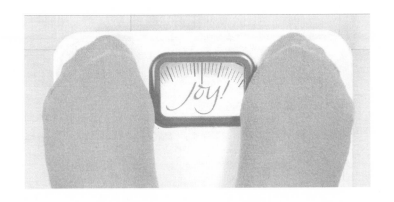

PART TWO

Scale Guidelines

CHAPTER 8

Using the "Right" Scale

You might think that weighing yourself is as simple as looking at the number on your scale. But you can't always count on the accuracy of the readout. Instead, many factors influence what the scale says before you even step on it. One of the most obvious is the quality of your scale.

Excellent cooks know they can often improve a dish by using the correct size pan, the right temperature, and the proper amount of intensity when mixing the ingredients. In the same way, to get the most from your scale, you need to follow a few guidelines that will give you the most accurate numbers.

Start with the Best Tool

Remember the old style of scale with the round dial? Maybe you still have one of those in your bathroom. That type of scale might be just fine, but if it's 20 years old, you're probably seeing a lot of variation that's not related to what you weigh. If your weight number bounces around a lot, I suggest you consider getting a new scale.

Some companies still offer analog scales, including ones with round dials. But most of the scales sold today use digital technology. Overall, these appear to be more accurate, but even a high-end digital scale can give you inconsistent readouts.

How to Test Your Scale

To test the accuracy of your scale, start by placing it on a hard surface rather than a carpeted floor. Then step on and off the scale five times in a row. You should see the same number at least four of those times. If you get several different readings, you need to look for a new scale.

Over the past few years, a lot more scales are able to provide accurate readouts for individuals with high weight requirements. If you know your starting weight is quite high, look for a scale that can accommodate your size and give accurate readings in the higher range of numbers.

Today, there are many consumer scales that can measure weights up to 400 pounds. But if you think you weigh more than that, consider visiting a hospital that offers weight-loss surgery. There, you will usually find a professional scale that measures a greater range of weight numbers.

The Right Scale

If we could find a scale that was perfect, it would make this part of losing weight so much easier. Unfortunately, there is no "god" scale. Most consumer scales lack the precision to be 100% accurate every time you step on them. Even an expensive model or a scale in the doctor's office can be out of calibration, resulting in inconsistent readings.

Recently I had a big shock at my doctor's office. It was 9:30 in the morning, and I'd had only a few cups of coffee and a small breakfast. But when I stepped on the scale as requested, it read seven pounds higher than my early morning weight at home!

Which reading was correct? The one on the doctor's scale or the one in my own bathroom? Actually, it doesn't matter. Weighing yourself on five scales will give you five readings. And in reality, even if two of them match, it doesn't mean you are seeing the "right" one.

Only One Scale

In the process of becoming friends with the scale, you may need to cut off a few outside relationships. Once you have a good scale at home, or you've chosen a place to weigh yourself, make that the only scale you ever get on.

No more jumping on the scale at your mother's house or testing the one at your health club just for fun. If you are visiting a friend and you notice a scale in the bathroom, ignore it! Don't step on it out of curiosity to see how it compares to yours at home.

Make an agreement with yourself that, even though it's tempting, you will not scale hop. Remember, your goal is to become healthy about this part of your weight-loss journey, not reinforce your obsession with weighing yourself.

Buying a New Scale

You don't need to spend a lot of money to get a good scale. In fact, some of the least expensive ones are more accurate than the high-end ones.

Start by deciding what's most important to you. Do you want lots of features or simply a scale that shows your weight? A basic one will give you a weight readout and that's all. For me, that's plenty of information. I don't like the idea of adding a lot more details to my weight monitoring.

But if you love gadgets or like the idea of seeing a lot of numbers, a complex scale is fine. Here are some of the features available on newer scales:

* **Talking scale**

  First thing in the morning, I certainly do not want a scale to loudly announce my weight. But if you like hearing the numbers out loud, go ahead and get this type of scale. A talking scale can also be helpful if you have limited mobility or poor vision that makes it hard to see the numbers on the readout.

* **Body fat measurement**

  Many popular scales calculate weight, body fat, hydration levels, and even your income. (OK, maybe not that last item.) But many of the currently available scales promise details on every aspect of your body. If you love data, this might be your dream scale.

I'm not a huge fan of these scales because they tend to be inaccurate, or they give inconsistent results. I also question whether the extra details provide any useful information.

I've had clients tell me their complex scales simply made them more obsessed about the measurement numbers. Over time, your weight number, how your clothes fit, and how you feel physically will tell you more about your progress than a detailed body scan.

❖ **Scale with a memory**
Some newer scales come with an internal memory that tracks your own weight as well as the details for several different people. This might be useful if you are monitoring trends or you don't want to record your weight numbers. Personally, I don't need the scale to remind me of yesterday's weight.

I believe the best tool for most dieters is a reliable digital scale that gives you today's weight number and nothing more.

Be sure to check out the Special Report titled *How to Buy a Reliable Scale*, which is included in the free support materials for this book.

www.FriendsWithTheScale.com

CHAPTER 9

What Affects the Scale

*D*id you know that the barometric pressure or high ocean tides can influence the numbers you see on your scale? Or that stress can make your body refuse to lose weight?

I'm sure you've had times when it seemed as though your scale had gone crazy. Some days, for absolutely no reason, your scale number will bounce around like a ping-pong ball. Or your weight will suddenly drop several pounds when you haven't changed anything in your routine.

Other times, the scale will act stuck or arbitrarily show a higher weight than the day before. Occasionally, in spite of your best efforts, the scale will just do whatever it wants.

When your scale gives you a strange readout, remind yourself to be patient and wait it out. Within a few days or perhaps a week, your body will settle down, and you'll see a more accurate measurement of your weight.

Here are 14 factors that can affect what your scale says. Some are things you can change to get more accurate scale readings. But many of them are totally out of your control. Whenever your scale seems to defy logic and show numbers that don't make sense, consider whether your body might be reacting to one or more of these issues.

Factors with Lots of Control

1. **Time of day**

   You'll always get the most accurate and consistent scale readings with an early-morning weigh-in, before eating or drinking anything. Weighing late in the day can show numbers that are two to four pounds higher than a morning reading.

2. **Water intake**

   Drinking lots of water doesn't actually improve weight loss. But it does increase your body's efficiency and it helps remove the byproducts of fat metabolism. Because water intake affects your body's fluid levels, it may help the scale move more consistently.

   When you don't drink enough water, you can become dehydrated, which forces your body to retain fluids as a way of protecting itself. Surprisingly, this can show up on the scale as an *increase* in your weight!

3. **Routine exercise**

   During the initial recovery phase after an exercise session, your muscles pull in water to help them recover. Sometimes this spills over into the next day or two. You may notice a higher reading on the scale the day after you've done a vigorous walk, bike ride, or exercise class.

4. **Extra-hard exercise**

In spite of what you've seen on popular weight-loss TV shows, killer levels of exercise don't always result in a drop on the scale.

When you push yourself extremely hard at the same time you drastically cut calories, your body protects itself by conserving resources, including fat stores.

If you notice your scale number either getting stuck or going up after a series of hard workouts, decrease your exercise intensity for a week or two and see if that helps budge the reading on the scale.

5. **Stress**

High levels of stress keep your body on alert in case it needs to suddenly jump into battle. To stay prepared, it protects itself by holding onto every last resource it can find. This translates into fluid retention and unwillingness to release fat stores.

If your weight appears to be stuck, consider whether you are going through a high-stress time. Unfortunately, any time you're dealing with intense stress, you may have difficulty losing weight.

Factors with Some Level of Control

6. **Travel**

   As you already know, most people retain fluids after any type of travel, including bus or train as well as airline trips. Changes in atmospheric pressure or even local weather conditions can affect scale readings by several pounds in a day.

   While this is especially noticeable after an airplane trip, a driving vacation can result in a similar problem. When you ride in a car for a long time, blood tends to pool in your lower legs. Eventually, this causes fluid retention and an increase in your scale number.

7. **Hormone changes**

   Along with making you feel bloated or puffy, PMS, menopause and other hormone fluctuations can cause fluid retention lasting seven to ten days. Some women continue to retain fluid the first few days of their periods, keeping the scale reading artificially high.

8. **Changes in muscle mass**

   Here's a common myth—muscle weighs more than fat, so that must be why the scale is up. This is partly true because, over time, building more muscle and improving strength does affect body weight. But it takes several months of consistent exercise before you'll see weight changes caused by an increase in muscle mass.

When you challenge your muscles with strength training, your body pulls extra water into the cells. Initially, this can show scale changes that are unrelated to your fat stores.

9. Extreme temperatures

In hot, humid weather, your body tends to puff up and hold extra fluids. To check this out, turn your rings on a hot, muggy afternoon and notice how puffy your fingers have become.

10. Barometric pressure

When the barometric pressure drops, such as when a storm is approaching, your body may retain fluids more than usual. If you live near the ocean, you may notice a similar effect during times when the tides are high or fluctuating a lot. These weather-related issues are especially common for individuals with arthritis or other conditions that respond to weather changes.

Factors with Almost No Control

11. Illness

When your body is fighting an illness, it protects itself by conserving resources until you feel better. A bad cold or the flu can temporarily slow your weight loss while your body attempts to recover and repair itself.

If you have the stomach flu or other conditions that causes vomiting or diarrhea, your body will typically pull in extra fluid to try to get back in balance. So even though you might see a major drop in your scale number, you're not getting an accurate picture of changes to your fat stores.

12. Medications

Many types of medications affect how your body metabolizes fat stores. In fact, blood pressure or diabetes medications can cause your body to become very stubborn, making weight loss difficult.

Any time you take antibiotics or do asthma treatments, your system may temporarily hold on to weight. When your body decides that it's safe to release extra weight again, your progress will improve.

13. Chronic physical conditions

Long-term treatments for conditions such as diabetes, arthritis and lung problems can cause a range of frustrating side effects. With many of these health issues, it's common to experience weight gain or the inability to lose weight in spite of being faithful to following your diet.

Steroid medications nearly always cause weight gain as well as make it difficult to lose weight. Many treatments for cancer or heart conditions are also potential culprits in the dreaded weight gain.

14. Surgery or physical trauma

When your body perceives that something traumatic has happened, it will grab onto every resource it can find to help it heal and recover from the assault. But in the process of doing this, it retains fluid, sometimes a lot of fluid. Unless there's a medical reason such as being on diuretics, it's never wise to weigh yourself right after a major surgery. You'll only see a reflection of the fluid level changes inside your cells.

Body trauma from things such as a fall or an auto accident will affect your weight in a similar way. To heal bruises and other soft tissue injuries, your body rushes extra fluid and nutrients to the areas that were harmed. Again, if you jump on the scale, you'll probably see an increase in the number simply because of shifting fluid levels.

Patience Required

So there you have it. Now you can understand why the number on the scale can bounce around so much or even be off by several pounds. Learn to recognize times when your weight might be affected by one or more of these 14 factors.

When you're dealing with any of these factors, stay patient and wait a few days. Before long, you'll probably see a different scale number that's much closer to your true weight.

CHAPTER 10

Scale Myths and Beliefs

W hen Helen arrived at my office, she looked angry and upset. As she stomped over to my office chair, she practically shouted at me.

> *I don't understand the scale at all! I've been on a very rigid diet plan for the past six days. But when I got on the scale today, instead of my weight going down, it was actually UP one pound. I concluded that my diet was not working, and I headed out to a fast food restaurant for a double cheeseburger and fries.*

When you've been perfect but the scale doesn't move in the right direction, do you typically give up on your plan? If so, it's time to recognize that sometimes the number on the scale has *nothing* to do with your dieting efforts.

One of the big mistakes dieters make is to assume when the number on the scale goes up, it means they've gained weight. Most of the time, this is simply not true.

Often, what you see on the scale is not even related to your actual fat stores. Instead, you're observing a host of interior body changes that affect fluid levels inside your cells.

Common Scale Myths

You've already learned about 14 different factors that can affect your scale reading. But sometimes you want to see progress so badly that you grasp at anything that seems to indicate you could be losing weight.

Here are a few of the most common myths about the scale.

❖ **You can lose weight with the flu.**
   "Wow! I lost twelve pounds last week when I had the stomach flu." Even if it looks as if you've lost that much, curb your excitement. You didn't actually change your fat stores during the time you were sick. You just shuffled your fluids around.

   Vomiting or diarrhea will usually bring a drop on the scale. But your body simply did a major fluid dump, and after a few days, it will shift in the other direction.

   Even a respiratory flu with fever and cold symptoms doesn't cause a weight loss. Maybe you've said, "The only good part of being sick was that I didn't eat anything except soup and gelatin for almost a week. So at least I've probably lost some weight."

Sorry, your body doesn't work that way. If you go without eating much for a number of days, your body clamps down and holds onto its resources. So even if the scale number drops, it's probably not true weight loss.

❖ **I'm gaining muscle.**
Maybe you've thought, "I've been working out a lot, so that must be why the scale is up." Since you know that muscle weighs more than fat, it's easy to assume you've simply added scale weight due to having more muscle.

But here's the kicker. It takes a minimum of eight to 12 weeks before this shows up as a true change on the scale. After only a couple weeks of lifting weights, you're still observing fluid level changes, not an increase in muscle.

❖ **It's from the cupcake!**
Each morning Debbie jumped on her bathroom scale. But lots of days, she would weigh herself again right before going to bed. On days when she'd eaten extra food or sweets, she believed the scale would immediately reflect her "mistakes."

"See," she would exclaim. "That's because of the cupcake I ate this morning!"

You probably know it doesn't work that way. It takes a lot longer than a few hours for your body to turn extra calories into fat stores that register on the scale.

❖ **You're doing it all wrong.**

Over the years, lots of diet plans have laid out strict rules that are supposed to help you lose weight more effectively. In fact, you may be led to believe that the scale isn't changing because *you are doing something wrong.*

Some programs tell you to combine food groups or eat certain foods only at specific times of day. Others suggest you avoid eating any carbohydrates after mid-afternoon.

Several recent books recommend you alternate "fasting" days with higher-calorie-intake days. These authors and programs aren't giving out bad or dangerous advice. And if you follow their suggestions, you probably will see a drop in the numbers on the scale.

But in a lot of cases, people lose weight because they cut their total calories, not because of a magical food combination or an unusual eating pattern. In the long run, most of these approaches are not practical, and as a result, people eventually slide away from following them. Unfortunately, in a short time, the "lost" weight comes right back.

Does the Scale Keep You Motivated?

When I was a young child, my mother fastened a tape measure to the back of our family room door. About once a month, she would have me stand next to the tape, then lay a ruler on top of my head and determine how much I'd grown since the last measurement.

Since kids grow in spurts and stops, it was common to have many months go by without any changes in my height. Now suppose my mother had become frustrated with the lack of results and angrily stomped out of the room, saying, "It's not working. No matter how hard I try, you're just not growing. Since you aren't getting any taller, I think I'll just quit feeding you."

Of course, she never did this. Most people understand that changes in a human body take time and not seeing results doesn't mean things aren't happening. But sometimes we forget this, and after trying so hard to lose weight, we stomp off to eat a bag of cookies because the scale hasn't moved.

If you believe the only way you can stay motivated is to see results on the scale, you'll probably struggle with making progress. Any time you hit a plateau or the scale doesn't change for a week or two, there's a good chance you'll give up because "it's not working."

Instead of letting the scale determine your actions, switch to a new belief. Remind yourself, "If I stay motivated, of course I'll see results."

This approach takes more effort because we tend to be impatient and we want to see things change quickly. But weight loss works the same way as the measuring tape on my family room door. It requires lots of patience.

Cultivate a new belief that your efforts are paying off even when the scale doesn't show any change. Then trust that if you stick with your plan, you'll eventually see the outcome you want.

Don't get discouraged if your weight doesn't show changes every week. Remember, weight loss is never a straight line. If you get impatient, you may give up on your efforts just when the scale was ready to move.

Power Key 3: Focus on my actions, not the reading on the scale.

CHAPTER 11

Seven Scale Guidelines

*F*or many years, Paula lived with a scale obsession that often left her feeling depressed and hopeless after weighing herself. Then she decided to disconnect from all of the crazy thoughts and behaviors she'd struggled with for so long. Instead, she began thinking of her scale like an email. Each day, it gives her a little input. But once she steps off, she never gives it any more attention and mentally walks away from the numbers.

> *At my highest, I weighed 225 pounds. One day, I decided to take a whole new approach to managing my weight. I focused on healthy eating, moderate exercise, and finding new hobbies rather than doing mindless eating. I would do things like clean out a junk drawer rather than munch on chips in front of the TV. I learned to talk out my feelings rather than bury them under food. It took a couple of years, but I reached my goal weight of 158 pounds. The best*

part is that I've maintained that now for many years.

The scale wasn't always my friend. But I got sick of feeling dominated by the negative feelings I got whenever I didn't like the number. So I wrote out a simple plan and told myself it was how I would live the rest of my life.

Now I weigh myself every morning, right after I get up and use the bathroom. I always step on the scale naked so I don't have to worry about any variation based on my clothes. I also remind myself not to let the scale reading negatively affect my day.

By weighing every day, I have learned to recognize the patterns and fluctuations that come with normal life. I don't panic if the number goes up. But if my weight is up three pounds for more than two days in a row, I do a quick review of things such as my water intake, my eating patterns, and how much exercise I've been doing. Then I address all three of those things, and within a couple of days, the scale is usually right back down again.

You can reach a similar level of comfort with your weigh-in rituals. As you build a friendship with your scale, stick with a few simple rules and never vary from them. No scale games, remember? Just reliable ways to gather the data.

Seven Guidelines

To consistently get the most accurate picture of your true weight, follow these seven guidelines:

1. **Early morning**

   Jump out of bed, go to the bathroom, then step on the scale. Record your weight, then head to the shower or turn on the coffee pot. Because there are fewer variables affecting it, your morning weight will always be the most accurate as well as the most consistent.

2. **Only once**

   When you get on the scale, make note of the first number it shows. Then write it down or post it to your online program and be done with it. Don't get on and off the scale several times to see if the reading stays the same.

3. **Don't go back**

   After you've weighed yourself and recorded the number, put the scale away or leave the room. If you store your scale in your bathroom, train yourself to ignore it. You won't learn anything new by returning to it later in the day. In fact, any other scale readings for that day will give you odd or inaccurate information.

4. **Never at night**

When you weigh yourself in the evening, you aren't seeing a true measurement of your weight. Instead, you're seeing a reflection of your day's activities and how they affect your body.

Weighing yourself at night can easily become a form of punishment. You might even catch yourself saying, "Let's see how bad I was today."

There are a few exceptions to this rule. One is the required weigh-in at group meetings such as Weight Watchers, TOPS (Take Off Pounds Sensibly) or similar programs. But always remind yourself the only official weight is the one on your own scale in the morning.

You may also have a challenge with getting a morning weight if you work nights or have an erratic schedule. In this case, pick the time of day that works best for getting on the scale, then aim to stay consistent with that choice.

5. **Consider daily weigh-ins**

I know you've heard lots of advice about how frequently to weigh yourself. But when you have a history of weight struggles, the scale becomes one of your best tools for staying on track.

Research studies have shown that people who weigh themselves every day are more likely to lose weight as well as maintain their success long term. So if it works for you, make getting on the scale a daily routine.

6. **Create a personal plan**

   If weighing yourself every day pushes you into obsessive thinking, set up a plan that fits for you. Instead of daily weigh-ins, consider getting on the scale once a week. Just don't let this become totally random. To get the most accurate information, stay consistent by always weighing yourself on the same day of the week.

   You may want to avoid using Monday for your weigh-in day. Because weekends usually involve different types of foods or changes in your activity, a Monday scale reading may be less accurate than one later in the week. I suggest using Wednesday or Thursday for your routine weigh-in because those days are not affected by weekend behaviors.

   Choose your weigh-in day based on what matches your needs. For some people, weighing every Sunday works well because it feels like a good start to the new week.

   During stretches of time when you decide to stay away from the scale, I recommend you still weigh yourself at least once a month. Pick a specific day such as the first or the fifteenth of each month. Then put a reminder on your calendar to step on the scale that day.

7. **Stop avoiding it**

   As you know, it's easy to avoid the scale when you suspect you've gained weight. But over time, this behavior gets you into more trouble. Let your scale become a gentle tool, not a hammer that beats you up. By setting up your plan for how and when you will weigh yourself, you can avoid the scale dread that comes when you've stayed away from it too long.

Strive to follow these rules consistently, even through holiday seasons, birthdays, and high-stress times. By staying with these guidelines, you'll avoid nasty scale games as well as the sudden shock of seeing high weight numbers after a long break.

CHAPTER 12

Healthy Scale Talk

*W*hen you talk about changes on your scale, what do you say to yourself? Most people look at their scale reading and immediately proclaim they have gained or lost weight. Here's an example: "I ate a couple of cookies yesterday, and sure enough, this morning I had gained two pounds."

Logically, you know your body did *not* add two pounds of fat stores overnight. In fact, most times when the scale number goes up, it's not reflecting your fat stores at all. Plus, you can't conclude that your body composition has changed based on a single measurement.

Over a period of a couple of months, seeing a higher number on the scale probably does mean you've gained *some* weight. But you can't assume this after only one or two days of weighing yourself.

Change Your Scale Talk

Since you can't be sure if any number on your scale is permanent, don't automatically announce, "I gained weight this week." In your efforts to become friends with the scale, work on changing the way you talk about the numbers.

Here's a new way to discuss what the scale shows. Whenever you weigh yourself, you can say only one of these three statements:

* The scale went up.

* The scale went down.

* The scale stayed the same.

With all of these, you are reporting a fact, but you're not assuming the numbers indicate a true weight change.

When you refer to the scale reading this way, it helps you stay more neutral about the numbers. Instead of immediately feeling depressed because your scale reading changed by a couple of pounds, you remind yourself that this doesn't reflect a *true* number.

Fixing your scale talk may take time and effort. To help build your skills in this area, practice this new approach with friends and family members. You can even demonstrate it for your weight-loss counselor or program leader. Instead of commenting that you gained or lost weight, use the new terminology: "The scale went up" or "The scale went down." Your leaders will be impressed by your mature way of viewing the changes in your weight.

The Big Picture
If you get too close to your scale, you see only the tiny changes in the numbers, and you lose sight of reality.

When this happens, step back and get the bigger picture of your weight changes. Instead of staring at one or two numbers, create a visual way to demonstrate what's happening with your weight.

Lisa had struggled for years to manage her scale. But then she found a great way to change her attitude.

No matter how hard I worked at it, I couldn't stop weighing myself every morning. I tried dropping to once a week, but I just couldn't seem to stay off the scale for more than a day. Of course, I always went through emotional ups and downs based on what the scale told me. Intellectually, I know that the scale reflects water retention and other things, but I desperately wanted to see results every day.

After listening to my scale frustrations, my husband came up with a great solution, and we've both used it for years. We monitor a five-day and ten-day average. To help us do this, he created a spreadsheet that automatically calculates everything. So each morning, I put in the number the scale says, but I use my five-day average for my official weight.

Even if the actual scale reading is up for one or two days, it doesn't affect me emotionally because that's not my "real" weight. I've finally learned to love my scale

*for the tool it is. I know that if the average
goes up, I need to evaluate what's going
on and then change my behavior.*

How to Monitor Your Weight

Over time, you might find it helpful to see the bigger
picture of what your weight is doing. Here are some
ways to track what's going on with your scale numbers.

❖ **Make a graph to show your progress.**
Record your weight in a spreadsheet or chart,
then display it as a graph. Once a month, tape
your report to the wall, then stand back a few feet.
Notice how easily you can recognize the changes,
both positive and negative.

❖ **Track with a computer-based program.**
Dozens of online programs provide instant feedback
by showing a colorful visual of your weight tracking.
Seeing the big picture on your computer screen can
give you a much healthier perspective.

One of my favorite tracking programs is
the website Start Your Diet. I find the colorful
graphics on this site to be highly affirming and
motivating. To check out this resource, go to:
www.trackyourplan.com.

❖ **Monitor your body shape.**
Take body measurements at intervals such as once
a month. Don't make this complicated or get hung

up on your waist size. Instead of turning this into a math equation, plan on tracking only one number. Here's how to do it:

Measure the size of your chest, your waist, and your hips. Then add these numbers together for a single measurement.

Over time, track how much this number changes. Consistently seeing a decrease in the total number of inches becomes extremely motivating.

❖ **Your clothes don't lie.**
Keep a favorite pair of jeans handy, perhaps one that's a size too small. Every few weeks, pull them on and see how much closer you are to fitting in them. When you can fasten that pair easily, grab a smaller one. Each time your pants size changes, use the next smaller pair as a goal.

❖ **Ignore BMI charts.**
BMI, which refers to Body Mass Index, calculates a number based on your weight and height. I'm not a big fan of monitoring this because of the wording used to describe weight levels. Sometimes, BMI charts seem to shame people by labeling them as "obese" even after they've lost a lot of weight.

In recent years, some researchers have even challenged the BMI chart because they believe that, for many people, these designations aren't very accurate.

If you choose to track your BMI, keep in mind that it's simply another piece of data. Personally, I suggest you skip this tool and instead, use only three basic guidelines to monitor your weight progress:

* ❖ Your scale reading
* ❖ Your body measurements
* ❖ The fit of your jeans or your belt

As you continue to see improvement in these three factors, you can trust you are achieving a healthier body.

Power Key 4: Speak the truth—the scale went up/the scale went down.

CHAPTER 13

Who Owns Your Weight?

O ver the past year, Julia had lost almost 80 pounds. But to reach her goal weight, she still needed to lose a lot more. When she arrived for our weekly meeting, she sounded frustrated and upset. Here's what she said:

> *I am so tired of people asking me about my weight. From my family, my friends and the people I work with, I keep hearing the same questions over and over. "How much weight have you lost? How much do you still need to lose? What's your goal weight?"*
>
> *When I answer their questions, I don't usually get support or encouragement. Instead, I get raised eyebrows and unsolicited opinions about why I should use some other diet plan or special vitamin supplements.*
>
> *Lately, people are telling me that I'm getting too thin, and they wonder if I should stop losing weight. They seem*

*horrified when I tell them I still need to
lose another 40 pounds.*

*I think my weight-loss efforts should
be private, and I just wish people would
leave me alone. I don't want to be rude,
especially to my close friends or my
family. It's just that I can't figure out
how to avoid answering their annoying
questions. I'd like to come up with a way
to respond nicely but not have to explain
all the details.*

Everyone Wants Your Numbers

Like Julia, you've probably had times when you've
squirmed when being questioned about your weight-
loss numbers or your goals. And while you may not
mind people occasionally asking about your progress,
sometimes their questions feel way too invasive.

Regardless of your history or advice from others, *you*
own your weight. In fact, you own everything about it,
including your current scale number, your goal weight,
how many pounds you've lost, and how much you still
want to lose.

Even weight-loss professionals don't always manage
the numbers game very well. When Sandra took a short
break from her meal-replacement program, she went
through several days of having an upset stomach along
with severe cramps. Her program counselor actually
suggested Sandra was being punished for eating foods
not on her plan.

When someone tries to control you by taking charge of your weight or your numbers, take action immediately. Either challenge the person who makes the comment or walk away and protect yourself from this type of response.

Protect Your Ownership

As you claim ownership of your weight, you'll discover you don't have to give away information you'd prefer to keep to yourself. This includes every aspect of your weight-loss plan including how you're handling it and how well it's working. And unless you choose to share it, treat your weight number as a private detail in your life.

When Anne went through stressful times and gained a lot of weight, her husband decided it was his job to fix her. Over the next few years, he attempted to force Anne to lose weight by controlling everything about her.

Frequently, he would try to shame her by making comments to their friends about her being a "fat slob." He complained about her size and let her know that he found her weight totally offensive. Even worse, sometimes he would snatch food away from her in an effort to limit her calorie intake.

Instead of responding to his "help," Anne rebelled. Whenever her husband wasn't around, she would sneak food and eat huge amounts. Of course, her weight continued to climb. By letting her husband *own* her numbers, Anne never made much progress with losing weight or improving her health.

Building Ownership

So how do you avoid giving away ownership of your weight information, especially around pushy or demanding people? First of all, you need to take charge of your weight. Stop assuming you are required to answer questions about your weight numbers or your goals. Instead, learn how to respond in ways that protect your ownership.

Start by choosing which people you want to keep informed about your weight-management efforts. This might include carefully-selected family members and friends, and perhaps your weight-loss counselor. Even with these individuals, you don't need to give out all the details. Perhaps with your family members, you could share your weight numbers weekly or even once a month.

Remember, there's a lot more to your weight-loss picture than a number on your scale. Rather than only sharing your recent weight, let people know about all the ways you are making progress. Describe how you are handling food triggers or ways that you're motivating yourself to exercise every day.

Don't get caught in the trap of confessing every diet slip-up. Instead, focus on owning your actions as well as your goals. If you eat a candy bar instead of your apple, you don't have to announce it to the world. Food is not a moral issue and confession doesn't usually improve your weight-loss efforts.

What to Say to People

The next time someone outside your inner circle asks about your weight loss or your goals, give a generic answer. Experiment with simple phrases that avoid revealing specific numbers. Here are a couple of ideas:

* That's information I keep private.

* Outside of a few selected people, I don't discuss my weight numbers.

When someone asks how much weight you've lost, make statements such as "quite a bit" or "a moderate amount." You can also ignore the question and instead reply, "I've been making great progress. Thanks for asking."

If you continue to be pushed for an answer, use these responses:

* My weight-loss program teaches us to avoid talking about specific numbers. It can make us too obsessed and pull us off track.

* I prefer to keep the numbers to myself. But thanks for asking about how I'm doing.

When asked about your goal weight or how long you'll be on your diet program, dodge the question by saying, "I still have a little ways to go, but I'm doing really well at this point."

If you get tired of hearing people's opinions, including ones about whether you are getting too thin, blame your doctor. Most people respect guidelines and treatment plans from physicians. So you might say, "My doctor is monitoring my progress and wants me to stay on my program for a while yet."

Like choosing to wear a baseball cap to a social event, you don't need to explain or defend your actions. You own your weight, so it's your decision whether or not to tell people your numbers. If you prefer to keep the details to yourself, figure out ways to dodge the questions instead of sharing personal information.

Accepting Praise and Compliments

It can happen anywhere—the grocery store, a family reunion, a meeting at work. Someone practically shouts, "Oh, my goodness. You're so thin. You look fantastic." Or they offer sincere praise by saying, "Wow, you've been doing a great job with your weight loss. Congratulations!"

Even though it's nice to hear them, compliments can also make you uncomfortable. Often dieters will respond to a compliment by minimizing their progress. "Thank you, but I still have a long way to go." Or they'll talk about their struggles or the ways they aren't doing well at the present time.

If a friend approached you with a small gift-wrapped box, you would smile and reach out to graciously receive the gift. Think of compliments and praise in the same way. Even though you might squirm from the attention, simply accept the gift and aim to make the person feel great about having offered it to you.

When someone gives you the gift of a compliment, respond by exclaiming, "Thank you for saying that. I appreciate it so much. You really made my day!"

Then stop talking. Don't add, "But I've been really slipping up lately and I haven't lost much the past few weeks. It's been really hard." Sharing all of your struggles might help *you* feel better, but it decreases the value of the gift. Instead, graciously accept the compliment, thank the person, and move on.

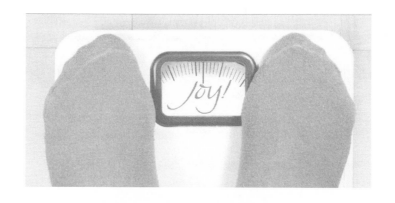

PART THREE

Scale Challenges

CHAPTER 14

When to Stay off the Scale

*W*henever Kathy goes on vacation, she leaves her diet and exercise program behind. She tells everyone she wants to relax and not worry about those things. But she always weighs herself as soon as she gets back home. "I need to know how bad I was, and the scale gives me an update."

Some dieters love punishment. When they return home after a vacation, they immediately jump on the scale to see how much damage they've done. "Oh my!" they shriek. "I gained eight pounds in two weeks!"

What nonsense! As you know, the scale number doesn't necessarily reflect your recent actions. While some people are capable of regaining weight rather quickly, most of what you see during these times is from changes in your body's fluid levels.

Even if you are totally comfortable with your scale, there are times you should *not* get on it, under any circumstances. If you insist on weighing yourself during these specific times, you are still a long way from being friends with your scale.

Five Times to *Never* Weigh Yourself

1. ### Vacations
    Right after a vacation, you'll nearly always see a false jump in your weight. In an effort to manage the challenges of travel, stress, and your mother-in-law, your body attempts to gather extra resources. This typically results in fluid retention, which increases your scale reading. But the higher number reflects the shift in fluid levels, not a true weight gain from added fat stores.

    Even simple changes to your routine can affect scale numbers. Eating new or different types of foods as well altering your exercise levels and sleep patterns can all cause fluid retention and a higher scale reading.

2. ### Holidays and celebrations
    Whether you're enjoying a holiday season or a small celebration for Easter or Memorial Day, special event meals will challenge your body's internal balance.

    Even if you don't think you ate too much at a holiday party or your mother's birthday dinner, be sure to allow your body a few days to get back to its normal balance. The same thing applies after holiday meals such as Thanksgiving. The "day after" is not the time to see how much you weigh.

3. **Travel**

   Any time you travel, you will probably retain water for a few days. This is especially true for airline travel, but it can also happen when you've spent long hours in a car or bus.

   If you travel frequently because of your job or for family visits, remember that even short trips of a few hours can cause you to retain fluids. Add in restaurant meals or snacks on the drive, and the next morning your scale number will probably bounce up a couple pounds.

4. **After you've been sick**

   Sometimes dieters get so desperate to see the number on the scale drop that they lose common sense. They are convinced that throwing up for three days will result in losing some fat stores.

   First of all, having the flu does *not* help you lose weight. In fact, the opposite is usually true. When you're sick, your body worries that it might need extra help to recover from the illness. Instead of giving up weight, it holds on tightly to all of its resources. That includes protecting your fat stores.

   Most people become dehydrated when they have the flu or some other illness. So again, remember that what you see on the scale is mostly a shift in your body's fluid levels.

Having surgery can cause even more drastic changes in your weight. Anesthesia, IV fluids, and pain medications all contribute to huge fluctuations in scale readings, sometimes showing an increase of even five to ten pounds.

Diagnostic procedures such as a colonoscopy can have a similar effect on your body. So unless you are taking diuretics or other medications that require close monitoring of your weight, stay far away from the scale for at least a week after any surgery or diagnostic tests.

5. **When you feel vulnerable**
    When you go through a crisis or a major loss, your confidence and self-esteem can disappear. Whether it's the death of someone close to you or the loss of your job, you need time to adjust and recover. Traumatic events such as the breakup of a relationship can leave you feeling empty and vulnerable for some time.

    Even having a bad day that includes extra food or alcohol can cause a temporary increase in your weight. Don't punish yourself for diet slip-ups by jumping on the scale.

    Any time you feel weak or vulnerable, postpone weighing yourself for at least a day or two. Instead of fretting about your weight, focus on healing and recovery. Stay off the scale until you get back into a healthy balance, both physically and emotionally.

The *Three-Day* Rule

Whenever you have a major shift in fluid levels, it takes your body a minimum of two to three days to regain its internal balance. Weighing yourself too soon will only tell you something about your fluid levels, not your true weight.

After a vacation, holiday, or illness, always wait at least 48 to 72 hours before you get on the scale. This gives your body time to settle down, rebalance fluid levels, and get back to a more normal status.

Although it's tempting to weigh yourself the morning after travel or holidays, getting on the scale will usually leave you upset. So build up your courage, and skip at least two or three days before checking your weight.

Follow the same guideline for special occasion meals that are out of your normal pattern. Even one birthday or anniversary meal can contain enough salt to make you retain fluids. After any unusual events, postpone your daily scale ritual for a couple of days.

In the same way, always give yourself a few days to fully recover from a bad cold or the flu before jumping on the scale. If you have an injury or surgery, you may want to wait as long as a week or ten days. By that time, your scale reading will show a far more accurate number than if you weigh yourself too soon.

Power Key 5: Wait three days to weigh myself after travel or holidays.

CHAPTER 15

The Dreaded Doctor's Scale

*M*argie hated going to the doctor. The biggest reason? The scale! Here's how she explained it.

> *At home, my scale is becoming my friend. But in the doctor's office, the scale is terrifying. I have to plan what I wear because I know it will become part of my "recorded weight." I also make sure to empty my pockets and not wear any heavy jewelry.*
>
> *One doctor's office keeps the scale in the middle of a busy hallway. Sometimes the staff members announce my weight loudly, which means other people can hear it. I wish doctors would think more about how it feels to be weighed in public, especially for a woman. It's one of my worst moments anywhere in life.*

Avoiding the Doctor's Scale

Most dieters agree that the most embarrassing place to get on a scale is at your doctor's office. For one thing, you are usually fully clothed and wearing shoes. Appointments are often in the middle of the day, so the scale reading is typically different from your morning weight.

For some people, an aversion to the doctor's scale becomes so strong that it keeps them from taking care of their health. Like most overweight people, Connie dreaded the doctor's scale. So, for many years she simply avoided going to her doctor's office.

> *I can't even tell you how many annual physicals and ob/gyn appointments I have canceled because I didn't want to face how overweight I was. I've been trying to stop risking my health because of my stupid fears about getting on the scale. But at the moment, I can't get myself past the dread.*

Even though physicians and their staff don't intend to humiliate their patients, many people can't escape feeling shamed and embarrassed about being weighed. Phyllis told me, "It feels like an invasion of my most private information. They don't make me take off my underwear in the middle of the hallway. But that's exactly how it feels when I'm told to step on the scale."

For some people, the doctor's scale seems like cruel punishment. It screams how bad you've behaved and asks why you can't seem to manage your weight better. But sometimes avoiding the scale can cause added risk to your health.

Until her recent heart attack, Angie had not gone to a doctor in more than 40 years. She said, "Being weighed at the doctor's office always made me cry. So even if I was sick, I wouldn't go to the doctor because I knew the staff would weigh me." How sad to let a metal object hold control over your life and your health!

Manage the Doctor's Scale

You may not realize this, but getting on the doctor's scale is *not* always necessary. In fact, most of the time a scale reading doesn't provide the physician with any critical information.

We know that certain health problems require close monitoring of body fluid levels. This includes heart disease and some types of cancer as well as being on medications such as diuretics. But if you're seeing the doctor for a bad cold or a twisted ankle, you may not have to be weighed.

The next time you go to your doctor's office, instead of automatically stepping on the scale, ask whether your weight is important for that visit's diagnosis or treatment plan. You might even explain you are working with a new program that recommends you stay in control by monitoring only a morning weight on your own scale.

The Magic Statement

Skipping the doctor's scale may be a lot easier than you think. Here is a simple line that has worked for me at many doctor's office appointments. When a staff member asks me to step on the scale, I say, "I prefer to not be weighed today. Is that okay with you?"

Interestingly, I've not had any of the staff members insist I get on the scale. They usually say, "That's fine." If you want to keep the conversation even simpler, just say, "I decline."

Even an annual physical shouldn't necessarily require that you be weighed. On the day of your exam, be sure you step on your own scale in the morning, then ask the doctor to record that number as your current weight.

To build up your courage for avoiding the doctor's scale, practice what to say ahead of time. Explain that you prefer to avoid using any scale except your own. Then say, "Here's what my weight was this morning. Feel free to write it in my chart."

You can also request to wait until after you've met with the doctor before getting on the scale. In many cases, you'll be able to skip it entirely or at least negotiate what gets recorded in your chart.

Barbara decided to help educate her doctor about her weight loss. First, she asked to speak with the doctor before being weighed. In the exam room, she began the conversation with her physician by saying, "Let me fill you in on what I've been doing the past several months."

Then she described her weight-loss plan, talked about all the things she was learning, and shared the amount of weight she had lost since the beginning of the year. The doctor was excited to learn about Barbara's progress and never did insist she step on the scale.

When You Can't Escape the Scale

I'm aware that Medicare and some insurance policies require that the physician obtain an accurate weight at every medical visit. So if you're informed that getting on the scale is required, here are three options to consider:

❖ Offer the scale reading from your early morning weigh-in at home.

❖ Step on the scale but close your eyes or stand backwards so you can't see the readout.

❖ Request that the staff member not tell you the number or say it out loud.

Regardless of how you negotiate with your doctor's office staff, avoid getting caught up in scale games. Instead of pulling out your thinnest pair of summer shorts or an extremely lightweight outfit, wear normal, comfortable clothes and leave your shoes on. This will reinforce your new belief about ignoring scale readings other than your own at home.

Most important, let go of your fear and dread before you enter the doctor's office. Then respond to the situation as an intelligent, confident adult. If you agree to step on the scale, avoid looking at the number or train yourself to ignore it entirely.

A bad week on your program certainly doesn't change your value as a person. When Candice realized how much power she was giving the doctor's office scale, she came up with a stronger way to manage it. She said, "I want to walk into the doctor's office feeling like a valid human being. Then I want to walk out feeling the same way. I've decided it's up to me to take charge of the scale and not let it decrease my personal value."

Managing Other Scales

What if you are participating in Weight Watchers, TOPS, or another plan that includes regular meetings or office visits? The protocol for most of these programs includes stepping on the scale at each meeting. How do you avoid letting the required weigh-in affect your new friendship with the scale?

Heather struggled with this a lot. During her weekly meetings at a medical clinic, she always dreaded getting on the scale. She lived in fear of having her weight number go up and being "scolded" by the staff for not doing a good job on her program.

Finally, she decided to change how she talked to the staff members. Regardless of her scale reading, Heather routinely began the conversation by saying, "Let me tell you about all the good things in my week." As she described her successes, her scale number became less important.

Although you may need to follow the rules set by your weight-loss program, you can still be in charge of how you manage the scale.

First of all, before you get to the meeting, think about your goals regarding the weigh-in and have a clear idea of what you want. When it's your turn to step on the scale, let the program staff know about your needs.

Here are a few ideas you might try that can work at almost any type of weight-loss meeting:

* Inform the staff person you don't want to know the number on the scale.

* Request to be told only whether your number went up or down from the previous visit.

* Ask if it would be acceptable to weigh at home instead of at the meeting or program office, and then share that number for their records.

Remember, *you* own your weight. While it's fine to get information from a program visit or doctor's scale, it shouldn't ruin your life. Instead of sinking into feeling shame, embarrassment, or humiliation, decide that *you* are in charge. Then manage the scales and numbers in your life with confidence and integrity.

CHAPTER 16

How to Retrain Yourself

When you've had a long history of struggling with the scale, you might be afraid that you'll mess up on your diet plan if you even go near one. In this case, you have a *thinking* problem rather than a *scale* problem.

As you work on becoming friends with your scale, you may need to retrain yourself on how to use it effectively as well as how to respond to the numbers.

Create New Beliefs

If you continue to believe the scale will ruin your life, it will. Instead of letting your actions be controlled by your scale, work on changing your beliefs. Trust me, this isn't as hard as it sounds. By focusing on how you *think*, you change what you *believe*.

Have you ever wrecked your car? If so, you probably had to build up your courage to get behind the wheel again. But by changing your self-talk about driving, you were able to create a new belief. You might have said:

❖ Driving again feels scary, but I can conquer the fear and trust that I'm safe.

❖ I'm a good driver, so I'll be fine with going to the store today.

❖ The more I practice driving again, the better I'll feel in my car.

These statements lead to a stronger belief than if you told yourself, "I'll never be able to drive again."

Changing your thoughts to create new beliefs also works with the scale. Let go of your fears and start building new messages around your scale numbers. Begin by telling yourself, "Of course I can become friends with the scale."

Then use one of these phrases to help strengthen your beliefs:

❖ I don't fear the scale because I know it's only data.

❖ If the scale goes up, that doesn't mean I can't manage my weight successfully.

❖ I can simply read the scale number, then walk away and have a good day.

Here's another way to let go of your old scale beliefs. Think of getting on your scale as being like the weather report. A forecast for rain doesn't tell you what kind of day to have. It simply tells you whether to take along an umbrella.

In the same way, if your scale reading moves up a couple of numbers, don't let it ruin your entire day. Just pick up your "healthy-living umbrella" and monitor your meals and exercise a little more carefully.

Breaking Up Is Hard to Do!

For years, Lori had been hooked on her scale and was afraid to be away from it. So even when she traveled, she always took her scale with her. One day we talked about ways she could let go of her scale connection and become healthier about how she used it.

First, I reminded her that fluid levels shift a lot when you're traveling, which can cause scale readings that aren't accurate. Because of this, carrying her scale with her might actually have been harming her weight-loss efforts. As a result of our visit, Lori decided to leave her scale at home when she left on her next trip.

A couple of weeks later, she sent me this note:

I want to fill you in on my battle with the scale and how helpful your scale training has been. On my recent trip, I decided to follow your advice and leave my scale at home. The day I left, I was short on time so I didn't even weigh myself that morning. That meant I had an extra day tacked onto the time without my scale.

When I got back home, I followed your rule of waiting three days before weighing myself to let my body readjust. I will admit, that was hard. All those

*days without a scale were making me
anxious and uneasy. I was feeling fat,
and I was afraid I'd be horrified when I
was finally able to weigh myself.*

*Guess what! When I got on the scale
after ten days of not weighing, I was
actually down a couple of pounds. I
am so glad I had trained myself on this
new approach. Now I'm working on
extending my time between weigh-ins,
and I may even try to stretch it to once a
week. Before our meeting, I would have
thought that was impossible, or that if
I didn't weigh every day, I'd be wracked
with anxiety. But after this learning
experience, I'm feeling a lot healthier
about my relationship with my scale.*

If you've spent years obsessing about the scale or
even avoiding it, it may take some effort to change your
beliefs. Start small by making a few changes, then build
on your success over time until, like Lori, you have a
strong friendship with your scale.

Use New Messages

You will always have times when the scale will still
bother you. But by renewing your beliefs at intervals,
you can prevent it from taking over again.

Practice mentally detaching from the scale by
taking control of your response to it. Immediately after

weighing yourself, fill your mind with positive, healthy messages. Here are a few examples.

❖ Every day I'm getting healthier and stronger.

❖ My actions (not the scale) will determine my outcomes.

❖ I don't need to see the scale reading move to know whether I'm on track.

If you haven't stepped on the scale for a while, you may need to ease back into it. Make sure you don't suddenly give your scale power because of what it says. Step on and note the data. Then step back off and go live your life. Your real world is still there, regardless of what you weigh.

CHAPTER 17

Scale and Weight-Loss Patterns

*W*hen you start a new diet or weight-loss program, you'll typically go through a "honeymoon" stage. Strong motivation and enthusiasm help you soar through the early days of your program, and you start to believe that "this time" it will work.

At the end of the first week on your diet, you hesitantly step on the scale. And usually you are rewarded with the news that you've lost a bunch of weight. You cheerfully step off and head to the kitchen for your protein shake or diet meal.

Does this sound familiar? If you're like most people, you'll see a significant drop in your scale weight at the beginning of any new dieting effort. As you watch your weight go down, you feel motivated to stay on your diet because, obviously, "it's working."

But after that initial weight loss, your body can do strange things. Even when you stay 100% on your meal plan and do things exactly the same as you did the previous week, your weight may change by only a small amount. Worse yet, in some cases, it might actually go up a bit.

96

By now, you're aware that what you see on the scale is not always a true reflection of your body's fat stores. It takes time to see the real changes in your weight. So how do you stay motivated and stick with your diet when the scale stops rewarding you?

During my work over the years, I've observed a wide range of weight-loss patterns. Here are some typical results, based on the type of diet plan used.

Traditional Diet Plan

With programs such as Weight Watchers or TOPS, counting calories, or following diet or recipe books, most people average losing around one to two pounds a week. Here's the typical change you can expect when you start this type of traditional diet plan.

* Week 1 – highest drop, between 2 to 5 pounds, or even up to 6 or 8 pounds

* Week 2 – a little slower, around 2 to 3 pounds

* Week 3 – a small change, sometimes only 1 or 2 pounds, or even no drop at all

* Week 4 and beyond – weight loss slides into a more consistent pattern, usually showing a drop of 1 to 2 pounds a week.

Meal Replacement Plans and Low-Carb Diets

Highly structured diet plans usually bring a very different weight-loss pattern. Examples of this type of program include meal replacement plans such as

Medifast, low-carb diets, and commercial centers such as Jenny Craig or SlimGenics.

* Week 1 – highest drop – often between 5 to 10 pounds or more

* Week 2 – a little slower, around 3 to 5 pounds

* Week 3 – a smaller loss of only 1 or 2 pounds, or even no change at all

* Week 4 and beyond – weight loss usually slows to around 2 to 4 pounds per week.

Meal replacement plans tend to give the fastest, most consistent results, with many dieters continuing to average between 3 to 5 pounds a week.

Jack is a 42-year-old male who weighed nearly 350 pounds. He decided to use the Medifast weight-loss program which included six meal replacements a day and no regular food. In 150 days, Jack lost 150 pounds. That's an average of one pound a day!

Although Jack's pace of weight loss was certainly unusual, I've observed similar results with other individuals who have a high starting weight. This is especially common during the first few months on this type of diet plan.

However, I encourage you to be cautious about advertising claims suggesting unrealistic levels of weight loss. While some dieters will consistently lose five pounds a week, it's unusual for most people to see this beyond the first few weeks on *any* diet.

Weight-Loss Surgery

Procedures such as lap-band or gastric bypass surgery usually result in an even stronger weight-loss drop than standard diet approaches. Because there are so many variables with weight-loss surgery patients, I have not included a listing of typical patterns.

If you are considering surgery or have already had a procedure, your physician or hospital staff will guide you on knowing what you might expect in terms of weight loss.

Factors that Affect Weight Loss

Regardless of the type of diet or weight-loss method you choose, these five factors will always influence your speed of weight loss:

1. **High starting weight**

   The more weight you have to lose, the faster it comes off, especially when you begin a new diet program. Like Jack, individuals who need to lose a hundred pounds or more will typically experience large drops in their scale weight during the early weeks on a weight-loss plan.

2. **Gender**

   Males will almost always lose weight faster than females. (I know, it's not fair!)

3. **Aging**

   Somewhere after age 45, many people notice they gain weight more easily and have a harder time losing than when they were younger. This seems to be especially true for women.

4. **Physical issues**

   PMS and menopause or other hormonal changes as well as chronic health conditions such as diabetes can make your body resist losing weight.

5. **Mobility**

   Regular exercise usually helps boost weight-loss speed as well as consistency. If you have limited mobility, you may struggle with a slower rate of weight loss.

It's Never Fast Enough!

If you're like most dieters, your speed of weight loss will never be as fast as you'd like. Unfortunately, you can't *make* your body lose at a faster pace. Even if you exercise extremely hard or severely restrict your calorie intake, your body will lose weight at the pace it considers safe.

Rather than getting hung up on trying to lose weight as fast as possible, focus on areas in which you have power. Stay committed to your plan and follow it day after day. In addition, keep building your exercise level and trust that, over time, your body will give you the weight-loss results you want.

CHAPTER 18

Tracking Reveals the Truth

Sandy was spending the day working on a computer project that required a lot of intense focus. Mid-morning, she felt a little hungry, so she pulled a large bag of almonds out of the cupboard. As she worked, she kept reaching into the bag for a few more almonds.

After a couple of hours, she finally took a break from her work. Suddenly she realized that she'd eaten more than half the bag of almonds. Then she read the label on the package and was horrified to learn those almonds had added an extra 900 calories to her daily total.

Does this sound familiar? When your scale won't budge, you may get discouraged and start questioning everything. "Am I doing something wrong? Do I need to use a different diet plan? Should I just give up on my goals?"

But maybe your stuck scale isn't related to any of these. Perhaps you're just not aware of some of your actions around food. When you get immersed in a project or activity, it's easy to slip into mindless eating and not even notice what you're doing.

Instead of quitting when you feel discouraged, switch your focus away from your emotions or worry. Instead, analyze the data. Go back to basics and review the details of your program to see if your estimated totals are still accurate.

Track Everything Again

For at least one or two weeks, meticulously record your food intake in your journal or online. Monitor everything you are eating to make sure you haven't let a few extra foods slip in.

Sometimes it's helpful to check nutrient details such as the grams of fat, protein, or carbohydrates you are taking in each day. To accurately separate your intake into these categories, look for an online program or software that automatically does this for you.

With meal plans that include a specific number of calories or carbohydrates, you might assume you've been matching your intake goals. Yet when you put everything into a computer program, you may be shocked to find that your numbers are a lot higher than you thought.

Here are my favorite online tracking programs. (See the Appendix for a full list.)

www.myfitnesspal.com

This free program works great for most people. It includes a mobile app that lets you scan labels on your cell phone and instantly get nutritional details on a food. The one downside to this program is that you have to put up with a lot of advertising.

www.trackyourplan.com (Start Your Diet Program)
For a small annual fee, this user-friendly program gives you an extensive food database and great charts and graphs as well as a built-in community of people who will encourage you on your journey. The site is totally ad-free.

www.weightwatchers.com
The easy-to-use online tracker for this program helps you see exactly where you are each day with your allotted points. I like the way you can create "favorite meals" so you need to add only one entry if you eat the same foods again.

Be Honest with Yourself

Don't skip recording certain foods because you're embarrassed you ate them! It's easy to trick yourself into thinking you're on track when you're actually padding the totals a bit.

Be especially careful with restaurant meals where you might "forget" to record the two pieces of bread or a dozen tortilla chips. Write it all down and face the calorie or point totals head on.

By separating your real actions from what you think you did, tracking makes you face reality. I've found this myself when I'm working on losing weight. Most days I'll assume I've stayed within the boundaries of my diet plan. But when I go online and record my intake, I'm usually surprised at my actual food totals.

When David first started to use a food journal, he kept two lists. First, he estimated the number of calories and fat grams he thought he'd eaten and jotted those numbers on a piece of paper. Then he used an online program to track his actual food intake. He also started measuring most of his foods to make sure of his actual serving sizes.

"I was shocked," he said. "I was way off on my totals in a lot of areas. For example, I thought I was eating one cup of breakfast cereal when it was actually twice that much. Because I don't cook, I didn't know how to estimate a cup of anything!"

Weigh and Measure Now and Then

Serving sizes have a way of increasing over time. It's amazing how a half cup of ice cream can grow until it fills a large cereal bowl. Every so often, recheck your foods to be sure they are matching your designated serving sizes.

Be especially vigilant with nutrient-dense foods that come in small pieces. Rather than take a guess at how many nuts equals one ounce, count out the exact number so you can stay accurate with your calorie totals.

Many diet programs urge you to record not only your foods but all of your thoughts and feelings each time you eat something. This helps you figure out the times when you are eating in response to your feelings or emotional needs. If you find this helpful, go ahead and track this much detail.

But if you're like most people, once you've tracked at this level for a week or two, you've probably gathered what you need to know. At this point, use your judgment on whether you need to continue to record this level of information.

Long-Term Tracking

Most people don't have to monitor their food intake forever. I suggest you track your foods until you no longer need to. Once you feel confident you are staying within the boundaries of your plan, just do an occasional checkup to verify the details of your food intake.

Here are three situations in which I encourage you to continue to track and record your actions.

* You easily lose your focus, and have found that tracking helps you stay consistent on your plan.

* Your program includes meetings with a staff person to review your record.

* You typically skip recording when you're off your diet or you've overeaten.

Based on what works for you, follow your judgment about tracking. But even if you dislike the effort required to monitor the details, go back to tracking once in a while to be sure you are accurately following your plan.

CHAPTER 19

Trouble in Scale City

*H*ave you ever been tempted to beat up your scale? A few years ago, Karen told me about how she got so frustrated with her scale that she destroyed it.

> *Like a woman possessed, I'd climb aboard the scale every morning, hoping to see that elusive number that would make me feel successful. Even though my dream weight was generally unrealistic, any slight variance from it would throw me into a full-blown bad mood.*
>
> *Eventually, I figured out there was a flaw in my own thinking. Every day, I was weighing myself as a success or failure as a person! Finally I got so tired of being jerked around emotionally by my scale that, after dark one night, I picked it up and carried it outside.*
>
> *I placed it in the middle of the driveway and ceremoniously beat it to*

*death with a six-pound sledgehammer.
The whole time, I kept yelling at the
top of my lungs that I was not going to
measure my value any more with one-
inch numbers on an LCD screen.*

*For months afterward, that battered
shell hung on my wall like a trophy deer
head. My new scale and I have a much
better, more balanced relationship now.
We check in with each other about once a
week to see how things are going. But now
it doesn't rule my day or shatter my heart!*

Like Karen, your bad emotional connections to the scale can go back many years, and often the memories aren't positive. Even after you've worked on building a healthier relationship with your scale, you may still have times when you'll struggle with it.

You know weight-loss success is not dependent on how you relate to the scale. But continuing to have a love-hate relationship with that little piece of metal or plastic can sabotage all of your efforts.

Scale Denial

Lucinda told me, "I have a mostly love relationship with my scale because the only time I weigh myself is when I'm on a diet program! The rest of the time, I avoid it entirely because I don't want to see what it says."

Like the old phrase, "See no evil," avoiding the scale can delude you into believing everything is fine. But if you weigh yourself only when you think you're doing well, you're probably in denial about what's really going on.

Suppose you fell off your diet, so you skip getting on the scale for a week or two. Then you reach a point where you're afraid to step on the scale because you know the number will have gone up. Weeks stretch into months, and you still don't weigh yourself.

Scale denial is simply thinking, "If I don't weigh myself, it's not happening." But eventually, this only makes your situation worse. The longer you ignore what the scale says, the harder it is to face the reality of your situation.

This is similar to not looking at your credit card bill when you've spent way more than your budget. Of course, facing the truth early on will help you pull in your spending and prevent the damage from getting worse. In the same way, monitoring your weight at intervals helps you see if you've been exceeding your food budget.

Courage to Weigh

If you've let yourself get caught in the scale avoidance trap, it's time to move past this roadblock. But as you know, becoming friends with your scale may take courage.

Here's a five-step guide for overcoming fear and denial, and then getting back on the scale.

1. **Pick a day.**
   Decide that you're ready to face reality. Pick a day in the middle of the week rather than a

Monday. Then plan to weigh yourself first thing that morning.

2. **Weigh and ignore.**
    On your chosen day, take a deep breath, get on the scale, then step back off. Ignore the scale reading and go about your day. If it helps, don't even look at the number.

3. **Do this for three days.**
    Repeat this weigh-and-ignore pattern for three days in a row. Don't give the scale number any power. Just ignore it.

4. **On day four, write it down.**
    By the fourth day of getting on the scale, you'll have adjusted to the number and moved past your fear. That's the day to record your weight.

5. **Add the next step.**
    Once you've reached this point with your scale, set up a plan for how you will manage it from now on. Choose the timing that fits best for you, weighing daily, weekly, or even once a month.

Weighing yourself after a long break requires courage and determination. But once you take that step, you move past a major barrier. After that, you'll be able to return to your goal of building a lasting friendship with your scale.

CHAPTER 20

Letting Go of Scale Memories

*L*ike many long-term dieters, Sharon despised the scale. She disliked seeing the numbers, and she hated how she felt every time she weighed herself.

When she first came to my weight-loss clinic, Sharon would stand backwards on the scale and ask me to record her weight but not tell her the number. She was fine with my stating whether the number had gone up or down, but she didn't want to know her true weight.

Sharon had been angry with the scale for many years, and she wasn't willing to let go of her feelings. She was also angry with herself for gaining weight. For her, hearing someone say the number out loud was embarrassing and demoralizing. So I agreed to let her manage the scale in the way she requested.

After several months of working together, I asked her what it would take for her to let go of her negative feelings and become friends with her scale.

Sharon thought for a minute, and then began to describe how her mother had always scolded her and berated her about her weight. Starting in grade school, she had been forced to get on the scale every week and was then chastised if her weight hadn't changed.

Sharon wasn't actually angry at the scale. Instead, she still felt resentful toward her mother for all the years she'd had to endure this "scale abuse."

After listening to her story, I asked Sharon, "Would you hate your car because someone criticized how you drove in your teenage years?" She laughed and said, "Of course not! But I guess that's what I'm doing with the scale."

Sharon had never thought about how strongly she was holding onto her childhood memories. Once she separated her feelings toward her mother from the weight-loss work she was doing, she was able to let go of her intense, negative feelings about weighing herself.

The next time Sharon arrived at the clinic, she took a deep breath and then stepped on the scale. But this time she faced forward, and after standing there for a few seconds, she announced her weight number so I could record it. What a great example of letting go of scale angst!

Shame and Embarrassment

In your efforts to become friends with the scale, you may have to face some old memories. Feeling shamed or embarrassed around being weighed can stick with you long past the event.

Tracy described an experience from her childhood that she's never been able to shake. When she was in the sixth grade, the teachers were instructed to weigh all the students who were assigned to their classrooms. Here's her memory of that awful moment.

> *I can still see the lavender dress with white trim I was wearing that day. My mom had made it for my Easter dress, using a pattern labeled for "chubby-size" girls.*
>
> *As each student took a turn stepping on the scale, I was horrified to realize the teacher was saying everyone's weight out loud. My weight was one-hundred twenty-six pounds, and to this day, that number still burns in my ears. I was so embarrassed and sad, mostly because I weighed more than almost everyone in the class, including the boys. Unfortunately, that picture and those words have never left my mind.*

Over the years, I've heard many similar stories of how being weighed in public left people feeling horrified or embarrassed. When she was in the seventh grade, Suzanne had a male teacher who announced each student's weight to the class. When it was her turn, the teacher not only said the weight number but added, "This one is a really big girl. She actually weighs more than I do."

Fortunately, most schools have eliminated the embarrassing ritual of weighing students in public. But for people who went through this type of humiliating experience, it can be hard to let go of those negative memories. At a subconscious level, you might still be recalling those awful feelings and assuming you'll have them again.

I encourage you to practice the skill of reframing your negative scale thoughts. That means when you flash to those memories from years ago, say to yourself, "Those old messages don't apply to me now. I am a strong, capable person, and I will continue to move forward in this area of my life."

Don't Shoot the Messenger

When you weigh yourself, acknowledge the numbers but don't blame your scale for your struggles. Being angry at your scale won't suddenly change your behavior and help you stay on your diet. In fact, scale anger usually has the opposite effect, causing the "screw it" response that leads to overeating.

In most cases, your weigh-in problems are not about the scale. Instead, you might be struggling with weak self-esteem, or you might have a fear of rejection if you aren't at a certain weight.

Remember, the scale is not your enemy. It's actually an important part of your weight-loss program. Train yourself to view your scale as an add-on to your diet plan as well as a tool for lifetime maintenance.

It's your decision whether to become friends with your scale or get rid of it entirely. Either one of these options can work. But straddling the fence between these two choices and hating your scale won't improve your weight loss or your life balance.

Make a clear decision about which way you will go, then face the scale reading as a healthy adult. Let go of past anger and resentment and, instead, build a relationship with your scale as a great weight-loss tool.

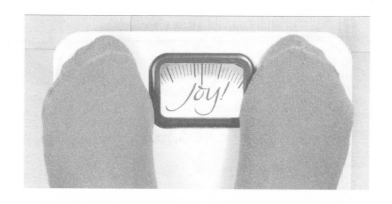

PART FOUR

Scale

Barriers

CHAPTER 21

When the Scale Won't Move

Suppose you've been perfect and didn't slip up on your diet even once. But when you step on the scale on your weigh-in day, it reads exactly the same as the week before. First you feel shock and surprise; then you get angry.

You can't believe it! It's not fair! You did everything right, but you didn't lose even one pound. At that moment, you may hate your body and feel convinced it has betrayed you.

Over the past week, you spent tons of time planning, cooking, and even sacrificing your fun. But now you wonder if you've wasted your efforts. You might even worry you'll never be able to lose weight.

Beth was a dieter who got frustrated easily. But in spite of this, she stepped on the scale every day so she could keep track of what her weight was doing. During one stretch on her weight-loss program, she became extremely upset because day after day, the reading on the scale stayed the same.

She said, "It drove me crazy! I couldn't stand the scale not moving, so finally, I made it move. I opened the refrigerator door and ate everything in sight!" Beth's scale weight certainly changed, but not in the direction she wanted.

When you give the scale that level of power, you usually end up regretting it. It's almost as if you punish yourself because the scale number won't move. That's like spending all the money in your savings account because the interest is too low.

The Totally Stuck Scale

We've all seen it—a stretch of time when the number on the scale absolutely will not budge! Every day you weigh yourself and it reads the same. Or maybe it bounces up and down a little but doesn't actually show any weight loss. And that's so frustrating.

No one knows exactly what causes weight loss to slow down. But at some point, this seems to happen to nearly every dieter. And sometimes, these frustrating stretches can go on for weeks or even months.

When the scale doesn't move, you begin to question everything you're doing. "Maybe I'm on the wrong diet." Or "I ate a cookie and that's why I'm not losing." Of course, both of these responses are incorrect. Instead, there's usually some type of physiological effect going on, and it's causing your body to hold on to weight.

If you respond to a stuck scale by getting upset or frustrated, you may unwittingly cause it to stay at that number even longer. As you know, stress signals your body to be cautious about giving up weight. When you get upset because the scale number won't change, you create a stressful event that might keep your weight stuck even longer.

The 30-Day Rule

In my work, I've learned that it takes approximately 30 days for your body to permanently shift weight as a result of a weight-loss plan. So when you've been dieting, you can't determine if your true weight has changed until 30 days have gone by.

If you're working hard to stay on your program, don't give up too soon simply because you see only a small weight loss. Stick with it for a solid 30 days, then compare your scale weight to where you were a month earlier.

In the same way, seeing your dream number on the scale doesn't mean anything unless you still see that number 30 days later. So don't assume you've maintained or avoided gaining just because the scale doesn't show any change in your weight.

Some years ago, I taught a weight-loss class that took place over the holiday seasons of November and December. In the first week of January, several class members were relieved because, in spite of holiday overeating and minimal exercise, their scale readings didn't show any weight increase.

But on the last day of January, some of these people were almost in tears. Their weight numbers had jumped several pounds, and it appeared the scale was firmly stuck at a higher reading. In this case, it took 30 days for the holiday eating to show up as changes in their bodies.

So back to the question—how do you cope with a scale that won't move? Most importantly, be patient and don't let your frustration cause you to give up on your efforts.

Often a change in your weight is just around the corner. When you give up because you think your efforts aren't working, you might miss the drop on the scale that would have shown up the very next day.

 Power Key 6: Never eat over frustration with the scale.

CHAPTER 22

How to Recognize a Plateau

*W*hen you've worked hard at staying solid with your diet and exercise plan, you expect to see your weight go down. And for a time, you may see a consistent drop nearly every single week. But occasionally, with no explanation, your scale number will refuse to budge.

If your weight stays the same for more than a week or two, you've probably hit a plateau. Researchers aren't sure why these slowdowns occur, especially when dieters have stayed completely faithful to a healthy weight-loss plan. And even though plateaus happen to nearly everyone who attempts to lose weight, hitting one can make you feel very frustrated and discouraged.

It's Not Your Fault, But...

When you experience a plateau, the tendency is to immediately blame your diet or your workout routine. In some cases, you may be right. Perhaps you unconsciously increased your calorie intake or backed down on your level of exercise.

But if you are confident that you haven't changed anything in your program, take a careful look at your routine. Sometimes your food intake will have crept up without you noticing it. When you actually look at your totals, you might realize you've been taking in a few hundred more calories each day.

Or perhaps the weather changed, and you had to cut your exercise time or eliminate part of your workout. Even small changes like these can affect your body and cause you to temporarily lose weight more slowly.

While no one can predict weight-loss plateaus, we know they are more likely to occur around certain times and circumstances. After you've been on a new diet for five or six weeks, your body adapts to the plan, sometimes causing a brief slowdown in your weight loss.

Whenever you're under a lot of stress or dealing with an illness or injury, your body tends to hold onto weight until it feels safer. So if you're experiencing a plateau, look for ways to let go of stress or anxiety. Even without making any other changes, you might discover your weight loss will pick up again.

The Halfway Point

Regardless of the amount you need to lose, your body seems to know when you're about halfway to your weight-loss goal. At this point, it's common to see a short period when nothing changes on the scale.

With people who have a high starting weight, a mid-point plateau can last anywhere from a few weeks to a couple of months. It's as though the body takes stock and reshuffles things. Then once it determines everything is in order, it cranks up the weight loss again.

At the start of his program, Gary weighed 398 pounds. Using a meal replacement plan, Gary watched his weight drop consistently, week after week. But right after he reached the landmark of losing 100 pounds, his weight loss stalled completely.

For three solid weeks, the scale number didn't budge. In spite of my encouragement and our discussion about plateaus, Gary was ready to give up on reaching his goals. But each week during our clinic meeting, I pushed him to stay focused and give it a little more time. Reluctantly, he agreed and stayed with his plan.

On the fourth week, he stepped on the scale at my center and almost shouted with joy. From the previous week's number, the scale showed a drop of nine pounds! With renewed hope, Gary continued on with his weight-loss plan and ultimately reached his goal of losing 180 pounds.

Weight Loss Is Not a Straight Line

As you know, your body is not a machine, and you can't predict how it will lose weight. When you start a new weight-loss plan, you'll probably see a fast drop in your scale numbers.

But then you may go several days or a week with no change at all. When this happens, it's easy to get upset and assume you're seeing a plateau. However, just when you're ready to give up on your plan, your weight will suddenly drop three pounds overnight.

If your weight has stayed at the same number for three or four days, don't assume you've stopped losing. A true weight-loss plateau lasts a lot longer than this. If several weeks go by without any changes in your scale number, then you can probably assume you're experiencing some type of plateau.

To determine whether you've hit an actual plateau or you're simply seeing a temporary slowdown, track your weight on a spreadsheet or chart so you can observe the changes over time. If possible, put your weight chart up on a wall, then step back so you can get a more accurate view. In most cases, you'll realize your weight is still following a downward trend, even if it has stayed the same for a couple of weeks.

Permanent changes to your weight don't happen quickly. In fact, sometimes your body will take several weeks to translate your efforts into actual changes in your fat stores. Research shows that in many cases, faithful dieters experience a brief plateau right before the scale shows a significant drop.

Don't let a period of slower weight loss pull you off track. Instead, stay patient, keep following your healthy eating and exercise plan, and trust that a change in your scale number is right around the corner.

CHAPTER 23

Ways to Boost Your Weight Loss

Plateaus can certainly be frustrating, especially when you're working so hard at staying on your weight-loss plan. But if you aren't careful, experiencing a plateau can derail you entirely and cause you to give up on your efforts.

If you think your weight loss has slowed down a lot, go back to monitoring your food intake for a few days or a week. Use a tracking program or a calorie count book to recheck everything. That way you can see if the actual calories listed for your food items are matching what you think you've eaten.

Strive for Accuracy

Marty was proud of his new, healthy eating plan. He'd heard that avocados were an especially healthy food, so he started adding them to his salads. One day, he pulled out his calorie count book and was shocked to learn that he was adding several hundred calories, along with a lot of extra fat grams, to his salad each day.

"I'm really disappointed," he said. "I thought that avocados were good for us." I quickly reassured him that avocados are a very healthy food. But like other high-fat foods such as nuts, you have to limit them when you're trying to stay within a tight calorie range.

With almost any diet plan, you'll be following a set of standard guidelines. But don't ignore some of the basic principles that influence how fast you lose weight. Sarah described how she got caught on a common food issue. She had been carefully tracking her calorie intake each day, and she thought her totals were accurate. Here's how she got in trouble with her plan.

> I use an online program to make sure I'm within my nutritional goals. But recently I realized I was forgetting about a couple of food items. One of them is the half-and-half that I put in my coffee.
>
> One day, I calculated that my coffee creamer was adding more than 200 calories to my day, and I hadn't been putting that in my food log! After that eye-opener, I cut way back on the amount of creamer I use. I also make sure I include it when I record my food intake.

Staying accurate is not the same as becoming obsessed about your diet. It's normal to have fluctuations in your daily calorie or nutrient totals. So don't assume you have to be perfect with staying on your plan. Instead, set up a budget range for your total calories or points.

For example, rather than aiming for exactly 1400 calories a day, set a goal of staying between 1300 and 1500 calories. Having flexibility in your total calories or fat grams will make it easier to match your budget.

Drink Lots of Water

In spite of what you hear from many diet programs, drinking lots of water does not cause you to lose weight. Instead, it helps your body be more efficient at getting rid of the byproducts of fat metabolism. Staying hydrated also prevents fluid retention that can temporarily affect your scale changes.

Sometimes adding more water to your day is all it takes to make the scale budge. Set a goal of drinking six to eight glasses of water every day. If that seems difficult, commit to drinking at least four glasses a day. You can always add a few drops of lemon juice or a non-caloric flavoring packet to help make it easier to increase your water intake.

Some dieters find it helps to drink a glass of water right before eating a meal. This fills some of the space in your stomach and can make you feel less hungry. As a result, you might find you can eat more slowly as well as do a better job of monitoring your food intake.

Be Consistent

Once you choose a calorie or points range that fits for you, strive to stay within those boundaries every day. The more consistent you are, the faster your weight will come off. Also, be sure you are eating at fairly regular times, not skipping meals, or being sporadic with your intake.

Recently several diet books have suggested alternating higher calorie days with lower calorie ones. However, there's not much scientific evidence that you'll lose more weight as a result of this method. I've also found that dieters quickly get tired of this approach or struggle because their low-calorie day often comes the same time as a family gathering or other social event.

Another dieting concept suggests that you take one day off from your program each week and eat whatever you like. In theory, this approach assumes you won't feel as good after your "freedom day," and eventually you'll change your eating habits.

This sounds good on paper. But it has never worked for me personally or for my clients who have tried it. And overeating every seven days doesn't usually result in long-term success.

Skip the Slow-Downs

Alcohol in any amount, even one glass of wine or a beer, alters the way your body manages weight loss. It's kind of odd that alcohol works this way. You may think you're simply swapping those calories for something else such as a fruit or vegetable.

But for many people, drinking alcohol can slow down weight loss by as much as one or two pounds a week. So if you depend on an alcoholic drink to help you relax or enjoy a social setting, you may need to find a new solution.

For managing social events, consider drinking club soda from a wine glass or a diet soda from a highball glass. These options give you the feel of a drink glass in your hand, but after a few minutes, you'll hardly notice you're not drinking alcohol. The best part is that people around you will probably never realize you've made the switch.

Move a Lot, but Not Too Much

Generally, exercise will boost your metabolism and help speed up your weight loss. But doing the right amount is critical. I can't give you an exact formula, but I encourage you to listen to your body and strive for a moderate level of exercise each day.

Attempting to use extra hard exercise to force your body to lose weight faster will usually backfire. If you aren't taking in the number of calories your body thinks it needs to manage your exercise level, it will simply slow down and conserve resources, resulting in slower weight loss. Or you'll find yourself feeling hungry and then you'll be tempted to grab easy snacks that can skyrocket your calorie totals.

Extra Caution Required

If you're on a commercial meal replacement program such as Medifast or Optifast, you may need to pull back even more on exercise. The low-calorie level of these plans can't support an intense degree of exercise, and if you push too much, your weight loss can slow down or even stop.

During the first few weeks on this type of plan, your body struggles to maintain efficient energy delivery for exercise. Until you've completed the first month on a meal replacement program, limit your exercise to 15 to 20 minutes a day of gentle activity such as walking.

Eventually your cells become more efficient at using fat stores as an energy source and your body can handle stronger amounts of exercise. But during the entire time you are using a meal replacement plan, limit yourself to 45 minutes of aerobic exercise a day.

If you push your body too hard on this type of program, you may have a hard time recovering after your workout. Overly strenuous exercise can cause fatigue that lasts for several hours or even into the next day. You might also feel a lot hungrier than usual and notice more cravings for carbohydrates.

No Marathon Training

Don't push yourself on endurance activities or attempt to train for a race while you are on a meal replacement plan. Your calorie totals are simply too low to support this type of exercise intensity. Pushing too hard also increases your risk for health problems or injuries. The most discouraging part is that, in spite of your low-calorie intake, you may not lose much weight.

With any weight-loss plan, keep your workouts at a gentle level, especially during the beginning of your program. And if the scale numbers aren't moving in the right direction, drop down to an easier workout. Along with decreasing the risk of injury, you may also prevent yourself from getting tired of exercise and stopping entirely.

CHAPTER 24

Switching Things up with Exercise

M ary Ann had a great walking routine. At 6:30 every morning, she laced up her workout shoes and headed out the door. She followed the same route every day and walked at a moderate pace for exactly 30 minutes.

She also stayed on a healthy diet plan, and because she was a creature of habit, she ate almost the same thing each day for her meals. But after two months of not seeing a change on the scale, she was furious. "How can this *not* work?" she asked. "I'm doing everything right!"

And she was. When I reviewed her food records, I could tell she was averaging between 1200 to 1400 calories a day. She'd already lost 45 pounds, so her plan had been effective for some time. But she was still 30 pounds away from her goal, which I thought was a realistic one.

I suspected that her body had completely adapted to her daily exercise and eating patterns. So we decided to make some changes in her routine to wake up her metabolism and push her body to let go of weight again.

We started with her exercise plan because it was the easiest thing to change. Instead of a daily walk, we switched things up by having her ride her bike some days, then use exercise equipment at the gym on other days. On the days she did her walks, I suggested she alternate a fast, hard pace with a slower, gentler one.

It worked! Without making any changes to her food plan, Mary Ann was able to shake up her body, and she began to lose weight again. The new approach helped her stay motivated and optimistic, and within a few more months, she reached her goal.

Switch Everything Around

If your scale has stalled or you can't seem to budge off a plateau, you may have slid into a similar pattern. Your body has an amazing ability to adapt to a routine, and eventually it stops giving you the results you got in the beginning.

When this happens, you probably don't need a different program or a new personal trainer. Sometimes simply changing a few parts of your workout is enough to kick your body back into weight-loss mode. Here are a few things to work on.

* **Split your activity**
  Divide your usual routine in half, then split it into two different activities. For example, instead of walking 30 minutes a day, drop the time to 15 minutes. Then ride a bike or use exercise

equipment such as an elliptical trainer or a stair machine for the other half of your workout.

❖ **Vary the speed**

Whether you use an exercise machine or take a daily walk, you probably slip into going about the same pace every day. Eventually your body can predict exactly what you're going to do, so it adapts to the daily pattern.

To change this, intentionally alter the pace of your exercise. When you are walking, use a short, quick step for a while and then switch to a longer stride for part of your workout. If you're on a machine such as a treadmill or exercise bike, select a program that automatically changes the speed for you.

The same concept works with any type of exercise, including running, biking, or swimming. Simply changing your pace may be enough to wake up your body and get things moving again.

❖ **Fast/slow plan**

Alternating between different speeds will also boost your outcomes. Start your workout by walking for five or ten minutes. After you're warmed up, run for a short time, then go back to walking again.

Start this routine slowly by running for only 30 seconds to a minute, then dropping back to your regular pace for two to three minutes.

Repeat this sequence several times, gradually increasing the running part of your workout. You can do a similar pattern using a bike or any piece of workout equipment.

Change the Type of Exercise

You probably have a favorite type of cardio activity, such as walking or using a specific exercise machine. But in your efforts to shake things up, look at what else might fit for you and your body type.

As an alternative to your routine walk, consider bike riding or swimming. Or locate a gym or fitness center that has a variety of exercise equipment and try out some new machines. Experiment with doing five minutes on the stair machine, then hopping on one of the exercise bikes.

Even switching between outdoor walking and using a treadmill can wake up your body. When you set your treadmill at a pace of three miles an hour, it forces you to walk at precisely that level.

Try varying the speed at intervals or raising the elevation a couple of degrees to add a fresh challenge to your routine.

When you walk outdoors or on an indoor track, you unconsciously alter your speed at intervals. So maybe all it will take to boost your weight loss is to switch from a treadmill to an outdoor walk.

Manage Stress and Emotions

Did you know that your moods and emotional state can cause your scale to be stuck? You already know that high levels of stress will sometimes make your body hold on to weight. The same thing is true of depression and anxiety.

If changes to your exercise routine don't budge your weight, take a look at your emotional health. Plan to get a massage or do some relaxation exercises to help calm your body as well as your mind.

You might even talk with a counselor or a life coach to come up with better ways to cope with your emotional challenges. As you relax and let go of tension and anxiety, your weight might suddenly start to drop again.

CHAPTER 25

Jolting the Scale with Interval Training

*I*f your weight seems completely stuck and the scale number won't budge, it might be time to bring in a more drastic approach. We've already talked about several of the safe ways to shake things up, such as adjusting your calorie level and monitoring your totals more carefully.

But if your body has truly adapted to your exercise routine, I suggest changing the intensity of your efforts by using interval training.

First of all, you need a way to monitor how hard you are working during your exercise program. Of course, you can use a heart rate monitor or other device. But the easiest way to assess your workout is to listen to your own body.

How hard does it feel to *you*? In other words, what is your perception of how hard you are exercising? This approach, called "perceived exertion," simply has you evaluate how you feel at different points during your exercise routine.

Many personal trainers recommend the nationally recognized Borg Scale of Perceived Exertion. With this tool, you rate your exercise intensity on a 10-point scale that ranges from very, very light to very, very hard. This approach might be fine for athletes who are aware of small differences in exercise levels. But I've never liked this scale because, for most people, it's too complicated and hard to use effectively.

Easier Way to Measure Exercise

Here's a much easier way to monitor how hard you are working out. This simplified scale draws on only three levels of perception, so it's a lot easier to figure out the intensity of your exercise efforts.

To understand how it works, think about how well you slept last night. You could certainly tell me whether you slept great, woke up a lot, or perhaps slept hardly at all. You certainly don't need to choose between 10 levels of sleep to analyze your night.

In a similar way, you can use three levels of perceived exertion to rate how hard you are exercising:

* ❖ Easy – gentle, light exercise
* ❖ Moderate – feels moderately difficult
* ❖ Hard – sweating level, requires considerable effort

To use this scale when you are exercising, begin by warming up for five minutes at the Easy level. Increase to a Moderate level for the main part of your workout, then end with a cool-down period at the Easy level.

Be sure to listen to your body and use your own perception of how hard you are working out. Plan to stay at a level that feels moderately intense but not exhausting. As you lose weight and your fitness level improves, you can begin pushing yourself to the Hard level for short periods. Eventually your cardiovascular system will become stronger, allowing you to sustain this level quite a bit longer.

Another tool for monitoring your exercise level is the talk test. During either a Moderate or Hard exercise level, you should still be able to carry on a conversation without gasping for breath. At the same time, if you can still sing, you are probably not working out hard enough. Of course, if you couldn't sing before, this test may not work for you!

Interval Training

Now that you know how to monitor your exercise intensity, you can add interval training to your workout. Most of these programs teach you to alternate between short bursts of a hard exercise level and a calmer, more normal level. According to research, interval training burns additional calories, increases metabolism, and improves heart rate recovery.

While there are many ways to incorporate intervals into your workout, I suggest you keep it simple. And before you start, be sure you're ready for this level of intensity. If you have doubts, hold off on how hard you push during the high activity levels.

As you probably know, the goal of aerobic exercise is to challenge your heart rate and, over time, strengthen your entire cardiovascular system. Keep in mind that the most important outcome is not how high your heart rate goes during exercise, but how quickly it returns to a normal level.

Here are two basic ways to do interval training using a walking program. You can easily adapt these methods to any type of aerobic exercise.

A Short and Sweet Approach

Taught by Jonathan Roche, creator of the "No Excuses Exercise System," this approach alternates three-minute challenges with one-minute resting levels. You can read more about this great online exercise program here: www.noexcusesworkouts.com.

Here are the basic steps to follow for this interval workout. You may want to refer to the three exercise levels (Easy, Moderate, and Hard) discussed earlier in this chapter.

1. Warm up by exercising at the Easy level for three to five minutes. You can walk, jog in place, jump rope, or do anything that gets your heart rate elevated. Don't overdo it here; just get your body moving.

2. Increase your exercise effort to Moderate and stay at this level for three minutes. Then drop back to Easy for one minute.

3. Repeat this two more times, exercising at Moderate for three minutes, then dropping back to Easy for one minute.

4. Push yourself a bit more now, and exercise at the Hard level for three minutes, then drop back to Easy for one minute.

5. Push even more to a level of extra Hard for three minutes, then drop back to Easy.

6. Cool down by exercising at Easy for at least five minutes.

This workout will take 30 minutes. If that feels too long when you're getting started, drop one or two of the intervals. Just be sure to do both a warm-up and a cool-down activity at the Easy level for a full five minutes each.

Long and Short Intervals

Here's another way to approach intervals. This works especially well when you are using exercise equipment such as a treadmill or elliptical machine.

1. Warm up for three to five minutes at Easy level.
2. Increase your exercise level to Moderate and stay in that range for nine minutes.
3. Increase to Hard level and sustain that for one minute.
4. Drop back down to Moderate and stay at that level for nine minutes before increasing again to Hard for one minute. Repeat that sequence of nine minutes and one minute a total of three times.
5. After the third time at Hard, drop to Easy and stay at that level for five minutes for your cool-down time.

Creating Your Own Interval Workouts

You can do intervals with nearly any type of aerobic activity including walking, running, biking, or swimming. On a treadmill, you can push your level by increasing the speed or by raising the elevation. When you start using interval training, do only one of these changes at a time, then add the second one when you have improved your endurance and fitness level.

Athletes who are training for competition can push themselves to extremely hard levels during interval training. But if you are overweight, you need to be sure to match the intensity of your workout to your current physical status. Always listen to your body when you are exercising. What seems like an Easy level for some people may actually be a Hard level for you.

As you lose weight, you'll continue to see improvement in how your body handles exercise. So keep working at this by challenging yourself at an appropriate level. You'll be amazed at how your exercise efforts will help your weight loss as well as your overall health picture.

CHAPTER 26

When Your Weight Is Totally Stuck

*L*aura was fed up with her stuck body! For the past three months, she had followed her food plan perfectly, averaging a daily intake of around 1100 calories. Her intense exercise workout included an hour a day of fast walking or biking along with a strength-training program. But Laura had 20 extra pounds that wouldn't budge, and she was ready to give up on reaching her goal weight.

In one of our meetings, she confessed she was tired of working out so hard, eating so carefully, and not seeing the weight changes she wanted. After reviewing Laura's food and exercise diary, I felt confident she was accurate with her tracking and that she wasn't underreporting what she was eating.

Conventional logic would say that Laura's exercise routine along with her restricted diet should have easily resulted in weight loss. But apparently, Laura's body had slowed down to protect itself from losing its critical resources. So I proposed a rather dramatic program that I thought might shake her body up and help her lose weight again.

Making a Drastic Change

I asked Laura to take a 90-day break from her current plan and instead to follow a very different approach. Here was her new plan:

❖ Increase her food intake to between 1600 and 1800 calories a day.

❖ Decrease her exercise time by at least half, perhaps even two thirds.

❖ Practice daily meditation, stress management, and other relaxation techniques.

Laura was scared to death. She exclaimed, "I'm afraid I'll gain a bunch of weight and then I'll be even more stuck."

I reassured her that it wouldn't be that drastic. "Yes, you probably will gain some, but I think you'll be able to get your body out of its rut and help it start losing weight again."

Laura thought about it, then agreed to make the changes to her plan. For the next three months, she continued to see me every other week, bringing her exercise and food journal each time.

During the first three weeks of her new plan, Laura's scale weight went up five pounds. After that, it bounced around some, but it didn't climb any higher. Over the next couple of months, Laura worked hard at staying within her new calorie range, while keeping her meal plan filled with healthy foods.

After 90 days of this new approach, we were ready to shake it up again. So we dropped her calorie totals back to between 1200 and 1400 a day. At the same time, I asked Laura to gradually increase her exercise level but still limit her workouts to 30 to 40 minutes a day instead of her previous hour-long bouts.

Almost immediately, her weight began dropping again. Three months later, she'd lost not only her 20 pounds, but also the extra five pounds she'd gained when we shook up her program.

For Laura's body to perceive it was safe to give up weight, we had to completely retrain her metabolism. Once her body had adjusted to her gentler routine, she was able to increase her workouts again and manage her weight successfully.

Extremes Don't Usually Work

Carol was a frustrated 43-year-old who was having trouble losing 40 pounds. So she decided the solution was to train for a half-marathon race.

Over the next few months, Carol severely cut her calorie intake at the same time she began doing long runs. Eventually she adjusted to her activity schedule and was able to work up to running the required 13 miles for a half marathon. But to her dismay, she didn't lose even one pound.

In my coaching work, I've seen many clients who decided that an intense exercise program is the answer to losing a lot of weight. Research, as well as popular TV shows, supports the theory that the harder you exercise, the more weight you will lose. Sometimes that's true. But other times, it can go the opposite direction.

If you're thinking about training for a race or competitive event, work on losing weight *first*. Don't attempt to use a training program to force your body to give up fat stores. When you push your exercise level at the same time you cut calories, your body simply holds on to all of its resources. As a result, you may end up not losing any weight at all.

How to Retrain Your Body

Instead of using a hard-core plan such as training for a race, focus on keeping your workout level and your food intake in a healthy balance. Here is a guide on effective ways to use exercise to budge stubborn weight.

❖ **First 30 days**

When you begin a new diet or weight-loss plan, take a gentle approach to exercise. Start with the easiest activity you can imagine, such as walking at a slow to moderate pace for only 10 to 15 minutes a day.

Never double what you're doing. Instead, gradually add more time to your workout, but do this only five minutes at a time. By the end of 30 days, strive for doing 15 to 20 minutes of exercise at least three to four days a week.

❖ **Second 30 days**

After the first month on your plan, you can start increasing your exercise intensity. But rather than extending the length of time of your workout, physically push yourself a bit harder. Increase the speed of your walk or bike ride. Also introduce more variation in your terrain, such as adding small hills or raising the elevation on your treadmill.

Hold this new goal for the entire month, never exceeding 30 minutes of cardio workout each day. If you feel ready to do more, add more days to your routine, gradually building up to exercising five to six days a week.

* **Next 30 days and beyond**
  After you've made good progress toward your goals, you might be tempted to push a lot harder and try to force your body to give up more weight. Don't do it. Instead, continue to take a gradual approach to adding more time and intensity to your workouts. For example, increase your exercise time by five minutes each week rather than suddenly jumping to a one-hour workout.

Until you reach your goal weight or a number that feels comfortable for long-term maintenance, resist the temptation to do hard-core exercise. Pushing yourself with intense levels of activity may simply cause your body to protect itself by holding on to weight rather than letting go of extra pounds.

Monitor Your Exercise Levels

Sometimes it helps to know how your body is responding to your workouts. Once you've built up your exercise program, consider using a heart rate monitor to establish whether you're staying in a therapeutic workout zone.

My favorite type of monitor straps on your wrist like a watch. Any time you want to check your heart rate, you touch a sensor on the device and hold it until the monitor shows a readout.

More advanced monitors include a strap that goes around your chest. A sensor inside the strap sends a continuous signal to the readout screen of a device. You can either wear the monitor on your wrist or fasten it to your exercise equipment where you can see it easily. At some health clubs or gyms with fairly new equipment, this type of monitor may even transmit the readout to the screen on your workout machine.

If you want to see how exercise affects your body as well as observe your improvement, a heart rate monitor will be a helpful addition to your weight-loss program.

But while it's useful for some people, continually monitoring your heart rate may seem inconvenient and not that important for you. In that case, don't worry about using a monitor. Instead, listen to your body and simply pace your exercise at a moderate level.

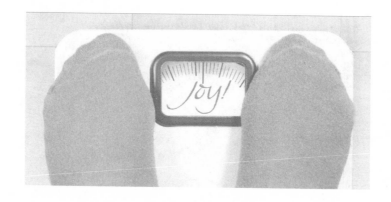

PART FIVE

Scale

Friendships

CHAPTER 27

Building the Friendship

*B*y now, you've learned a lot about the scale, including how it works and what the numbers really mean. Now it's time to take action and truly build a strong, lasting friendship with this weight-loss tool.

Maybe you're still having doubts about doing this. Even with all you've learned, you might still be thinking, "I can *never* be friends with my scale." But holding onto a love/hate relationship with it doesn't help you manage your weight.

I'd love to see you view your scale as a kind, understanding friend, but I also understand if you can't reach that point. If you're feeling uncomfortable with this, go back to Chapter Four and take the scale quiz again. Be sure you get clear about your own needs and whether you should keep your scale or throw it away.

Once you've made a decision that you will keep your scale, you have only one good option: *Commit to becoming best friends with it for life.*

Michelle is a Weight Watchers leader who lost 40 pounds quite a few years ago. She told me it took a while, but she finally learned how to be comfortable with her scale and see it as a good friend. Here's how she describes her scale routine.

> Every day, I weigh myself on my home scale. Then I record that weight on a calendar that hangs in my bathroom right above the scale. I also make little notations about my life. For example, I went out for Mexican food, did Pilates, hiked, etc.
>
> I have maintained this daily ritual for over six years, and it's been very helpful for me in maintaining my weight. If the number starts creeping up, I don't make a big deal out of it. I just write a notation as to why it might be up, and then I watch my behaviors a little more closely. It feels great to go back through the calendars and see where I was this month a year or two ago.
>
> The scale also gives me great accountability. My husband can see my weight chart, and if he notices my weight is up, he's less likely to suggest Chinese food for dinner. Instead, he might invite me to go on a hike or a bike ride. It's such a relief to be at a place of "friendship" with my scale. It doesn't control my life or my moods the way it did years ago.

The Dot Calendar

You probably have your own system for monitoring your weight. But if you'd like a great visual tracking system, consider using a Dot Calendar.

First, buy a set of green, yellow, and red stickers or stars. Next, find a wall calendar with large squares for the dates. Or go to www.100DaysChallenge.com and print off several months of the Dot Calendar.

At the end of each day, ask yourself, "If I lived every day exactly the same as this one, would I be likely to lose, maintain, or gain weight?" Then put a sticker on your calendar, using the following criteria:

* **Green sticker – Weight-Loss Day**
  Green stands for a solid day on your program. You stayed on your diet plan, perhaps did your exercise, and you managed temptations and food triggers well.

* **Yellow sticker – Maintain Day**
  Yellow means caution, or that your day could have gone better. Maybe you did a little extra eating along with no exercise. But in general, it was still a good day.

* **Red sticker – Gain Day**
  Red indicates you had a poor day on your program. Perhaps you had extra snacks, alcohol, or dessert, and you probably skipped your exercise plan.

As the weeks go by, keep putting stickers on your calendar to track your efforts. At any time, you can easily monitor your progress or struggles by counting the different colored dots. If you keep having lots of yellow or red dots, you're probably not going to see much change in your weight.

A couple of years ago, I went back to using the Dot Calendar to track my own weight-loss efforts. But instead of hiding it in the drawer the way I usually did, I tacked the calendar up on a wall in our closet.

After I'd had a particularly difficult week, my husband said, "I'm sorry I've pushed you to go out to restaurants where it's hard for you to stay on your diet plan. I feel responsible for all the yellow and red dots I saw on your calendar this week."

I loved getting that kind of encouragement and support. It also helped us change our restaurant patterns, and soon I started to see a lot more green dots on my chart.

Create a New Ritual

How would you like it if one of your friends always scowled fiercely before greeting you? That certainly wouldn't feel good to you. So why would you do that to your scale? In your efforts to become friends with this tool, you may need to change the words you say or how you think as you step on the scale.

Learning how to treat your scale better is not that difficult. Starting today, create a new pattern that you will follow each time you approach the scale.

First of all, no scowling or dirty looks. Instead, say "Hello" to your friend in a nice way. Then have a little chat about how things are going. Make note of the useful information your scale friend provides, then go about your day in a positive frame of mind.

Don't step onto your scale and beg, "*Please* reward me today!" Remind yourself that the scale gives only data. It does not tell you whether or not you are a good person. It also doesn't reflect how well you stayed on your diet plan yesterday.

Conversations with Your Scale

You might even talk to your scale and say something like, "Hi, Mr. Scale. How are you today?" You might even put "smiley face" stickers on your scale to remind you it really *is* your friend.

If your scale could speak, here's what it would love to say to you. "Welcome! I'm glad you're here today. And I'm so glad you are choosing to follow a healthy lifestyle! Let's work together on this to help you reach your goal weight and then stay close to that number for a long time."

Sometimes your scale will even acknowledge your struggles. "So... I see you've had a hard week (or month, or year). I can help by being a powerful tool in your program." Other times, your scale might give you wonderful praise and feedback. "Congratulations on making so much progress with your goals!"

When you've lost a bunch of weight, allow your scale to remind you it was *your own actions* that changed the numbers. Your scale would love to say, "You've made wonderful progress as a result of your efforts. And you did the work! All I did was hold up the mirror."

Set up a Long-Term Plan

Don't ask your scale to tell you about your life. Instead, focus on your day-to-day actions and trust that, over time, it will reflect the benefits of how you are living.

When you faithfully stick with a healthy living plan over the weeks and months, the odds are you will see positive changes in your weight. And if you aren't seeing the numbers you want, don't blame the scale. Simply evaluate your actions again, then figure out where you need to make changes that will move you toward the outcomes you want.

CHAPTER 28

Best Friends for Life

*Y*ou've done it! You've become friends with your scale. You've also changed your attitude and your thoughts about what the scale says. Now you treat the numbers as data, not judgment. And you recognize the weight you see on the scale is a reflection of many factors, not just your fat stores.

The biggest change involves what you say to yourself each time you get on the scale. You no longer let your scale punish you after a dinner party or a vacation. Instead, you allow the scale to remind you of your goals. Even when you've had a hard time with managing your weight, you don't let your scale become the target for your frustration.

When you're tempted to hate your scale, you remind yourself that it's only reflecting concerns about your behavior. This is similar to times when your weight creeps up and you loosen your belt or slip on a larger pair of jeans. When this happens, you don't hate your clothes. You know they simply reflect the changes in your body, and they help you recognize it's time to pay more attention to your actions.

Sometimes your scale will remind you to get back to your exercise program or to pitch that bag of cookies in the cupboard. When you are truly friends with your scale, you welcome these gentle messages and use them to support your weight-management efforts.

Preventing Scale Relapse

Right now you may be feeling confident about your relationship with the scale. You are determined to follow your new approach and never let the scale run your life.

But even the best intentions can slip away over time. So don't assume you'll never struggle with your scale again. Like any new skill, you need to practice treating the scale as your friend. You also need to be careful not to abandon this relationship when you go through a hard time.

To prevent scale relapse, stay committed to your new way of thinking, no matter what. If you struggle with your weight, don't put your head in the sand and pretend everything is fine. Instead, use the scale as a supportive tool to keep you focused on your goals.

Once in a while, let it provide you with a gentle reminder that you care about your health. Then focus on staying on track and continuing to manage your weight long term. Every single day, strive to live in a way that will make you feel proud of your efforts.

Your Lifetime Scale Plan

The final step in your new approach to the scale is to set up a clear plan for maintaining your friendship with it forever. First, I suggest you review the ideas in this book and pull out the ones that fit best for you. Select your top three or four tips, then use them to create a lifetime plan for how you will manage your scale.

My Lifetime Scale Plan

Use this quiz as a guide for creating your plan. Check as many answers as you wish.

1. I will weigh myself
   ___ Daily, no matter what's going on.
   ___ Daily except when I've been traveling, sick, or at a special event.
   ___ Once a week, on _____.
   ___ Once a month, on _____.
   ___ When I happen to think about it.
   ___ Never (because I've gotten rid of my scale).

2. I will track my weight by
   ___ Writing it on a paper record, a calendar, or a wall chart.
   ___ Recording it online or on a computer program.
   ___ Memorizing my current weight number.
   ___ Monitoring how my clothes fit.

3. I will manage the scale by
   ___ Weighing only in the mornings before eating or drinking.
   ___ Weighing only at my gym, health club, or doctor's office.

___ Not getting on any scale except my own.

___ Not weighing for at least 48 to 72 hours after travel, vacations, or holidays.

___ Not weighing myself at all.

___ Not having a scale in my home.

4. I will manage my emotional response to the scale by

___ Saying "the scale went up" or "the scale went down."

___ Reminding myself that it's only data, not a reflection on me.

___ Stepping on, stepping off, and leaving the room.

___ Focusing on my actions and my healthy behaviors.

___ Not weighing myself at all.

5. I will manage the scale at my doctor's office or medical clinic by

___ Saying, "I prefer to not be weighed today."

___ Asking to wait until seeing the doctor before getting on the scale.

___ Bringing a record of my recent scale weights at home.

___ Closing my eyes or standing backwards on the scale.

___ Requesting the staff member not to tell me the number.

___ Noticing the scale readout but completely ignoring it.

6. I will own my weight by

___ Telling people who ask that I don't wish to share specific numbers.

___ Saying I've lost "a lot" or "a bunch" rather than the exact number of pounds.

___ Sharing my weight numbers with only my family and selected friends.

___ Saying, "In my program, I'm not supposed to discuss numbers."

___ Graciously receiving compliments or comments about my weight loss.

Create a visual reminder

Once you've laid out your lifetime plan, follow it faithfully, year after year. You might find it helpful to post a summary of your answers in a place where you can see it often. Include reminders about each of these areas:

❖ Days and times you'll get on the scale and how often you'll weigh yourself

❖ Several examples of what you will say to yourself about your scale

❖ Reminders for managing the scale during unusual times such as travel or holidays

Even when you know your eating and exercise patterns might be causing your weight to go up, never abandon your friendship with your scale. Remember, your scale is a powerful tool in your weight-management plan. Use it faithfully as part of your lifelong commitment to healthy living!

Power Key 7: Smile at my scale and treat it like a friend.

☙ *APPENDIX* ❧

 Seven Power Keys for Staying Friends with the Scale
Use these messages as part of your positive self-talk.

Power Key 1: Never let my scale win!

Power Key 2: Remember that I can't trick the scale.

Power Key 3: Focus on my actions, not the reading on the scale.

Power Key 4: Speak the truth—the scale went up/ the scale went down.

Power Key 5: Wait three days to weigh myself after travel or holidays.

Power Key 6: Never eat over frustration with the scale.

Power Key 7: Smile at my scale and treat it like a friend.

For a printable version of the Seven Power Keys, go to:
www.FriendsWithTheScale.com

Resources Recommended by Linda Spangle

I realize there are thousands of weight-loss programs, books and resources available, but here is a list of my absolute favorites. Be sure to tell them I sent you.

Best Online Tracking Program
Start Your Diet
www.trackyourplan.com

This online program provides far more resources than most online tracking sites. It has an extensive food database that also allows you to add your own meals or food items. In addition to the tracking and connecting benefits, Start Your Diet includes the full text of my book, *100 Days of Weight Loss*, making it easy to stay committed to your goals.

The site also has an active online community with many categories of participants so you can find people who share your personal interests and challenges. When you post things on one of the message boards, many people will quickly offer personal words of encouragement or celebration.

Here's a quote from Start Your Diet owner, Chris Dziewulski:

There is a reason so many of our members are fans of Linda's work and make it an essential part of their day. Not only does she deliver great information and strategies, but the unique way she delivers that information into thought-provoking and retainable lessons sets it apart from other resources.

Best Online Exercise Program
Gentle Boot Camp for Overweight People
www.noexcusesworkouts.com

In this unusual exercise approach, Jonathan Roche and his online team walk you through a different 30-minute exercise program each day. You don't need equipment, just a pair of comfortable shoes and a great attitude.

The boot camp programs are all taped, so you can just log on to their website when you're ready, then follow the easy, encouraging instructions. The program focuses on interval training, which has been shown to greatly improve weight-loss results.

Author of *The No Excuses Diet: The Anti-Diet Approach to Crank up Your Energy and Weight Loss*, Jonathan is famous for his line, "Throw your rear-view mirror out the window!"

Best Online Support Community
Spark People
www.SparkPeople.com

Besides offering great instructional videos, articles and recipes, Spark People has one of the most active communities on the Internet. Whether you're working on losing more than 100 pounds or you're at the point of maintaining, you can always find people who share your areas of interest.

Type "emotional eating Linda Spangle" into the Spark People search box to find my forum and great resources for dealing with this difficult issue.

Best Weight-Loss Programs

Weight Watchers
www.weightwatchers.com

This program has offered a nutritionally sound support program for many years. But when you find a great leader, it can do wonders for your long-term success.

Michelle Malek, a Weight Watchers leader from Denver, Colorado, is one of the most dynamic people I've ever met. Her enthusiasm and encouragement have made a tremendous difference in the outcomes for hundreds of people. I hope you can find a similar, strong leader in your area.

TOPS Club, Inc. (Take Off Pounds Sensibly)
www.TOPS.org

TOPS meetings are held in local centers such as churches or recreation centers. Each meeting starts with members sharing challenges, successes or goals. The program emphasizes encouragement and support from other members along with inspirational content and awards for weight-loss accomplishments.

Here's a quote from TOPS president, Barbara Cady:

Since 1948, TOPS has been supporting thousands of members' understanding that they are far more than a number on a scale and that the scale is one of many tools that may be used in the weight-loss journey. We applaud the techniques illustrated in Friends with the Scale *for maintaining a healthy perspective as we work toward our best health.*

Quick Weight Loss Centers
www.QuickWeightLoss.net

This fantastic program provides a great model for running a successful franchise. Here's a note from Lynn S. Allen, Director of Quick Weight Loss Centers of Florida. She continues to produce one of the highest success rates in the company.

This book is a must read for every dieter who has ever had a love/hate relationship with the scale. Linda's practical tips make the weight-loss journey easier and more fun. I highly recommend Friends with the Scale *to all of our clients!*

Green Mountain at Fox Run
www.fitwoman.com

This wonderful weight-loss retreat center located in Vermont has been helping women develop a healthy relationship with food, exercise and body image for 40 years. Led by founder, Marsha Hudnell, this center provides an inclusive environment with several options for the length of your stay.

Private Weight-Loss Coaching
Linda Spangle, RN, MA
www.WeightLossJoy.com

In my coaching work, I help people tackle the hard issues such as emotional eating and other barriers to success. My popular one-year coaching program has brought success for many dieters who were totally stuck and unable to make progress with losing weight. With individuals who have completed this program, I've had close to a 100% success rate. Contact me at Linda@weightlossjoy.com for a free 15-minute visit.

Cookie Rosenblum, MA
www.RealWeightLossRealWomen.com

One of the most positive, encouraging coaches I know, Cookie believes that real weight loss, lasting weight loss, has to start from the inside out. She guides her clients toward moving beyond their barriers so they can focus on transforming their lives and having long-term success.

Cookie is the author of *Clearing Your Path to Permanent Weight Loss*, a workbook that guides readers on getting past the barriers that get in the way of success.

Sandy Livingston, RD, LD/N
www.Palmbeachnutritionist.com

From her office in Florida, Sandy provides weight-loss coaching both in person as well as by phone and online programs. She offers metabolism testing that can help dieters learn why they can't seem to make progress.

Melissa McCreery, PhD, ACC
www.TooMuchOnHerPlate.com

Author of *The Emotional Eating Rescue Plan for Smart, Busy Women*, Melissa provides coaching and programs for women who want to bring their A-game to their work and their life. Her clients discover the secrets to getting off the diet roller coaster and ending emotional eating and yo-yo weight loss. Her passion is helping women flourish as they create a lasting peace with eating and with food.

♔ ABOUT THE AUTHOR ♕

*L*inda Spangle, RN, MA, is a weight-management coach recognized nationally as a leading authority on emotional eating and other psychological issues of weight loss. She is the author of the award-winning books *Life Is Hard, Food Is Easy* (Lifeline Press, 2004) and *100 Days of Weight Loss* (Thomas Nelson, 2007).

A registered nurse with a master's degree in health education, Linda is a skilled teacher, counselor and writer. She is the owner of Weight Loss for Life, a healthy lifestyles coaching and training program in Denver, Colorado.

In addition to being interviewed by hundreds of radio shows, newspapers and magazines, Linda has been a guest on numerous TV shows including Fox News, Lifetime TV, and The O'Reilly Factor. She has been quoted in nearly every major women's magazine, including Shape, Redbook, Women's Day and O Magazine.

Linda is available for speaking engagements, training seminars and one-on-one weight-loss coaching. For information on her books and coaching programs, visit:

www.WeightLossJoy.com

www.DietCoachCafeBlog.com

Contact Linda at 303-452-1545, 1-800-298-3020 or by email to Linda@weightlossjoy.com.

Friends with the Scale
is also available in the following formats:

- ❖ ebook – www.amazon.com
- ❖ app – www.apple.com/itunes
  https://play.google.com
- ❖ audio – www.WeightLossJoy.com

❧ FREE MATERIALS ❧

Be sure to download the **free
support materials** for this book.

www.FriendsWithTheScale.com

- ❖ Tips for how to buy a reliable scale
- ❖ Interactive quiz to help you decide whether
  to keep your scale or toss it
- ❖ Interviews with leading experts in the
  weight-loss field
- ❖ Simple spreadsheet that automatically
  calculates five-day averages
- ❖ Guide for developing your lifetime scale plan
- ❖ Printable version of *Seven Power Keys for
  Staying Friends with the Scale*

Other Books by Linda Spangle
Available in bookstores, Amazon.com and www.weightlossjoy.com

Life Is Hard, Food Is Easy
The 5-Step Plan to Overcome Emotional Eating
This book will completely change the way you think about food, giving you a powerful strategy for conquering emotional eating and other barriers to your success.

You'll learn:

❖ How to get more control over food in your life

❖ Ways to manage emotions without using food

❖ How to get past sabotage, perfectionism and guilt

100 Days of Weight Loss
The Secret to Being Successful on ANY Diet Plan
These simple, day-by-day lessons will keep you focused and committed to your weight-loss program for a minimum of 100 days. This daily motivator will help you:

❖ Stay motivated all the way to your goal

❖ Learn instant tools that work in every food situation

❖ Make sense of meal portions, food triggers, and more!

The following pages contain an excerpt from the book *100 Days of Weight Loss*, showing you how easy it is to incorporate one lesson a day into your weight-loss program.

For more details or to purchase books, go to:
www.WeightLossJoy.com

☀ Day 1
I used to be that way...

You are so determined to make this program work. This time, you really want to stay on your weight-loss plan and reach your goal. But deep inside, you may be afraid you haven't changed at all and that you'll quit your program long before the 100 days are up.

Perhaps a tiny voice is reminding you of your past failures with dieting. In the beginning, you're always very excited and motivated. But after a few weeks, your enthusiasm drops, and without meaning to, you slip up.

Maybe you sneak an extra candy bar or a bowl of ice cream at the end of a bad day. Then you reason that, since you've already blown it, you can go ahead and eat more. Soon you get discouraged with your behavior and eventually you quit your diet completely, just like you always do.

Change your thinking

Stop right there! Your past does *not* determine your future. In fact, your previous failures have absolutely no effect on your ability to succeed now. Starting today, eliminate the belief that things *always* go a certain way or that you *never* stay with your goals. Whenever those doubts creep back in, immediately give yourself this new message:

I used to be that way, but now I'm different!

This powerful statement completely ignores whatever you did before and instead, it promises you can change your outcome entirely. Rather than being fearful that you'll repeat the past, build a new way of thinking.

Make up a new ending

Because *now you're different*, you can do anything. You can even create different endings for your old negative patterns. Suppose you've been worried because you "always gain your weight back." Come up with a new statement that describes what you can do to prevent this.

For example, you might say, "I used to give up on a diet after a few weeks. But now, I pull out my journal every day and use writing to keep myself on track."

When doubts creep in, remind yourself that *now* you handle life differently. Go ahead and invent entirely new outcomes for your goals, then remind yourself often about your ideas. Over time, these patterns will become permanent, and your dream of success will actually come true.

Today

* Make a list of any fears or negative behaviors that have hurt your weight-loss success in the past. Read each one out loud, and then say, *"I used to be that way, but now I'm different."*

* Then write new endings for them by completing this sentence: I used to _____ (fill in your old behavior), but now I _____ (write in your new ending).

* Read these new outcomes often, and then live in a way that makes them true.

☀ Day 2

Interested or committed?

Debbie was discouraged. "Whenever I start a new diet, I'm so determined to stay on it until I reach my goal. But after just a few weeks, something comes up—a party, someone's birthday—and next thing I know, I slip off my plan and give up."

Do you feel totally determined to stick with your efforts, or do you entertain a few nagging thoughts about "having fun" instead of staying on your plan? If you tend to start and stop every time you diet, you may want to look at the difference between being *interested* and being *committed*.

Interest slips away quickly

With *interested*, you tend to stay with your plans only until something better comes along. For example, you may decide that you're interested in losing weight, but when someone brings doughnuts to work, you quickly go off your diet.

When you're just interested in dieting, you depend on seeing results to keep you on target. So, as long as the scale keeps moving, you stay motivated. But if you hit a plateau or you don't see much progress for a few weeks, you may throw your program out the window.

Then, when you struggle, you blame everyone but yourself. You accuse your friends of ruining your diet because they eat potato chips in front of you. In addition, you fall into "if only" thinking, saying things like, "If only I had more time, more money, a new job, or a supportive spouse, then I'd be able to stay on my plan."

Committed means "no matter what!"

When you're truly *committed* to achieving your goals, you have an entirely different outlook. Unlike being interested, where it doesn't take much to detract you from your goals, being *committed* means you stick with it, *no matter what*.

Rather than depending on results to help you stay on track, you work on keeping your motivation strong, knowing that results will follow. You don't blame circumstances or other people for your struggles. Instead, you stay on your diet in spite of not having enough money, time, or supportive friends and family members.

Look carefully at your current efforts. If you tend to easily fall away from your weight-loss plan, decide if you're taking the *interested* approach. If so, strive for being *committed* instead. Start adopting a "no matter what" attitude, then convince yourself you can stay with your goals regardless of your daily challenges.

Today

❖ Decide that you will always be *committed* to your weight-loss plan, not just interested.

❖ In your notebook, describe how you will stick with your program, *no matter what.*

❖ Do at least one thing today that demonstrates you are truly committed. For example, take a walk or eat your vegetables—no matter what.

※ Day 3
Do it anyway

I don't feel like exercising today! Does this sound familiar? Then what happens? Do you push yourself and exercise in spite of not feeling like it? Or do you give in and hang out on the couch because you don't *feel* like making the effort?

Right now, you may be solidly committed to your goals. But what happens when you don't *feel* like cooking healthy meals or following your diet plan? If you aren't careful, you can easily slide back from being *committed* to just *interested*.

Committed means do it anyway

You don't usually wait until you *feel* like going to work. You just go. The same thing is true for visiting your mother or changing dirty diapers. Because you consider these things to be important, you do them regardless of how you feel at the moment.

In the same way, you don't have to feel like working on your weight-loss plan to stick with your program. To improve your commitment, learn to focus on your actions, not just your feelings. On days you're not in the mood for exercising or eating right, tell yourself to *do it anyway*.

Then skip the leftover cake and eat your fruit instead. Get up off the couch and put on your workout shoes. If you're really committed to your goals, you'll make these choices no matter what, regardless of whether you feel like it or not. Each day, take a few steps that will move you forward, even if you *don't feel* like it. Remember that when you're truly committed, you *do it anyway*.

Here's a summary of the differences between people who are *interested* in their goals compared to those who are *committed*.

People who are interested in losing weight
1. Stick with it until something better comes along.
2. Take action only if they "feel like" doing it.
3. Need to see results in order to stay motivated.
4. Blame people or circumstances for their struggles.
5. Easily give up when they face challenges.

People who are committed to losing weight
1. Stick with their plans no matter what.
2. Take action whether they feel like doing it or not.
3. Assume that if they stay motivated, results will follow.
4. Take responsibility for their own actions.
5. Keep going in spite of challenges and setbacks.

Today

❖ In your diet or exercise plan, identify a task you don't feel like doing, and then *do it anyway!*

❖ Notice how it feels to accomplish a goal by taking a "no matter what" approach to it.

❖ In your notebook, make a list of actions you plan to stick with today, regardless of how you feel at the moment.

⚜ Day 4
Boundaries, not diets

You've probably heard people say that diets are bad for you and that you should "never diet again!" In truth, the problem isn't usually with diets themselves, but with the rigid, perfectionist ways we use them.

If you're like most people, when you're *on* a diet, you try hard to follow it perfectly. Each day you strive to take in the exact number of calories, fat grams or carbohydrates allowed by the plan.

But if you slip up and eat a delicious (but forbidden) food, you figure you've blown it, so you might as well eat more. Soon you throw the entire diet out the window. This all-or-nothing approach never works because when you are *off* your diet, you cancel out the progress you made while you were on it.

Boundaries define your diet

Like it or not, to lose weight, you have to follow some type of system. Your plan can be quite rigid and meticulous, or as simple as deciding you'll eat less and increase your level of exercise. Instead of getting stuck on the word *diet*, learn to think of it as *boundaries* for your eating plan.

Picture your diet program as a road or a path. You can define the boundaries of your diet road based on the number of calories, points, or other factors you choose to follow. As you walk on the road each day, your goal is to stay between the sides of the road. Unlike strict or rigid diet plans, boundaries stay flexible. They provide guidelines, but at the same time, they allow for common sense and good judgment.

During times when you're strong and focused on your diet, you move the boundaries closer together, making the road narrower. When you take a break from your program or work on maintenance, you widen the boundaries and allow more variety in your plan. But even on a really bad day, you never eliminate the road or get off of it completely.

Set guidelines, not rules

Boundaries should give you benefits, not punishment! They should provide guidelines for you to live by, but not burden you with rules. You can define boundaries for any type of diet or weight-loss approach. Depending on your needs, you can simply adjust the edges of your plan to match where you are in life. By doing this, you'll be far more successful than if you punish yourself every time you step off the road.

Today

❖ In your notebook, draw a line down the middle of the page, creating two columns.

❖ Label one column "Narrow road," for your actual diet plan. Label the other "Wider road," for your maintenance or alternate eating plan.

❖ Under the titles, define your eating and exercise plans for each of these roads. Then decide on ways you can be flexible with them without losing sight of the healthy road you want to follow.

✺ Day 5
Magic notebook

Every night before going to sleep, Judy pulled out a spiral notebook and recorded her thoughts from the day. When she looked back over her progress during the past year, she concluded, "When I journal, I stay on track. It helps me catch the times when I'm slipping into emotional eating or getting discouraged with my efforts. Then I can make changes and correct these issues right away."

Get a "magic" notebook
For many people, recording personal thoughts or actions each day provides a lot of insight. It also serves as an outlet for emotions and struggles around weight-loss efforts. If you enjoy writing, experiment with tracking your thoughts and ideas around food and eating. Feel free to write as little as one sentence or as much as several pages.

On the other hand, if you don't find it helpful to write things down, don't force yourself to do this. But do keep a notebook handy as a quick tool for jotting down ideas about managing your eating patterns.

Eat it another time
Just because you think about a food doesn't mean you have to eat it. Whenever Jennifer got a craving for a specific food such as cheesecake, she wrote it in her notebook. She said, "By writing it down, I take it out of my head. I tell myself I don't have to think about it anymore because it's recorded and I can always return to it later."

When a food thought crosses your mind, remind yourself that you don't have to act on it. Instead, write down the name or even a description of the food, and then anticipate the pleasure of eating it sometime in the future.

Practice the skill of observing food cues, then letting them go. When you walk into a movie theater, notice the smell of popcorn, then forget about it. If it helps, record these cues in your "magic" notebook. Tell yourself, "That popcorn smells good, but I'm not going to eat any right now. I'll simply postpone it until another day."

Today

❖ Whenever you think about a particular food you want, write it down in your notebook.

❖ Plan that you'll eat it at another time. If you wish, add the amount you'll have and how often you'll fit it into your program.

❖ Stretch the times farther apart for eating this food. You may discover that after a while, certain foods don't seem as important to you as they once did.

LINDA SPANGLE'S
Websites

www.WeightLossJoy.com
Find details about Linda's books and weight-loss coaching programs as well as her extensive Media Room and contact information

www.DietCoachCafe.com
Linda's library of FREE training materials, audio programs and resources including the Weight Loss Mastery Program

www.DietCoachCafeBlog.com
Active discussions on current weight-loss issues as well as hundreds of FREE articles and resources

www.100DaysChallenge.com
FREE support materials for the book *100 Days of Weight Loss*. Includes 117-Page Journal, Quick-Start Guide, Special Reports, Tracking Charts, and a series of articles

www.TheDietQuiz.com
Based on your weight loss goals, age, body type and preferences, this quiz guides you to the diet that's right for you.